协和医学院系列规划教材

北京协和医学院精品教材立项项目

Concise Atlas and Laboratory Learning Guide to Human Parasitology

人体寄生虫学简明图谱与实验指导

主　编　王振生　王增蕾　魏春燕

主　审　王　恒

中国协和医科大学出版社

北　京

图书在版编目（CIP）数据

人体寄生虫学简明图谱与实验指导 / 王振生, 王增蕾, 魏春燕主编. -- 北京：中国协和医科大学出版社, 2024.10. -- (协和医学院系列规划教材). -- ISBN 978-7-5679-2341-6

Ⅰ. R38

中国国家版本馆CIP数据核字第2024PS7394号

主　　编	王振生　王增蕾　魏春燕
策划编辑	沈紫薇
责任编辑	沈紫薇
封面设计	邱晓俐
责任校对	张　麓
责任印制	黄艳霞
出版发行	中国协和医科大学出版社

（北京市东城区东单三条9号　邮编100730　电话010-65260431）

网　　址	www.pumcp.com
印　　刷	北京天恒嘉业印刷有限公司
开　　本	889mm×1194mm　　1/16
印　　张	7
字　　数	150千字
版　　次	2024年10月第1版
印　　次	2024年10月第1次印刷
定　　价	58.00元

Preface 前 言

在全球化浪潮和人们生活方式快速转变的背景下，寄生虫病的防治已成为公共卫生领域不可或缺的部分。人体寄生虫学作为医学领域内的一个重要学科，其学习对于培养高素质医学人才、提高寄生虫病防治能力具有极其重要的意义。鉴于此，我们精心编写了这本教材，旨在为临床医学、检验医学、护理学等相关专业的学生，以及广大临床医师和医学研究人员提供一本内容详尽、图文并茂、实用性强的参考资料。

本教材在编写过程中充分参考了国内外最新的人体寄生虫学教材，内容权威实用，精简易读，能够帮助读者轻松学习和掌握知识点和实验技能。本教材的主要特点如下。

一、结构清晰

本教材为便于学习，内容以实习任务的形式进行编排，全书共分为八次实习任务，每次实习任务将同类寄生虫划分在一起，内容涉及线虫、吸虫、绦虫、原虫、节肢动物。在每个任务内，内容按照寄生虫种类、实习目标、标本观察、标本示教、操作练习、课后小测、病例分析七个部分进行编排，充分满足教学所需。

二、内容全面

本教材涵盖了世界范围内主要流行的人体寄生虫40余种，尽可能收集了这些寄生虫不同发育阶段的高质量照片，多方面展示常见寄生虫的形态特征、实验操作技术等。

三、英汉双语

本教材采用以英文为主、中文为辅的方式编写，目的是提高读者的专业英语水平和学术交流能力，培养具有国际视野的医学人才。匹配的中文是为方便读者快速理解和掌握重要知识点而设置，言简意赅。我们相信，通过学习本教材，读者医学专业英语能力将得到显著提升。

四、实用性强

本教材既可作为高等医学院校人体寄生虫学实习教材，也可作为临床医师和医学研究人员的参考书籍。我们期望通过本教材的学习，读者能够更深入地了解常见人体寄生虫的基本形态、实验技能及临床应用，从而在实际工作中更好地应对各种寄生虫病问题。

本教材在编写过程中得到了国内多位资深寄生虫学专家的悉心指导和大力支持，他们的宝贵意见和建议为本教材的完善提供了重要保障。同时，我们也感谢所有为本教材出版付出辛勤努力的同仁们。

　　人体寄生虫学是一门持续演进的学科，新的研究成果和临床发现层出不穷。尽管编者力臻完善，但本教材难免存在一些不足之处。我们真诚地欢迎各位专家和读者提出宝贵的意见和建议，以便我们能够不断完善和更新内容，更好地为广大读者提供精准、全面的寄生虫学知识；为推动寄生虫学领域的发展、提高医学人才质量贡献一份力量。

王振生

2024年4月

Contents
目 录

Laboratory Rules ··· 1

Guide for Microscope User ··· 2

Practice 1　Nematode I ·· 4

Practice 2　Namatode II ··· 20

Practice 3　Trematode I ··· 28

Practice 4　Trematode II ·· 40

Practice 5　Cestode ·· 50

Practice 6　Protozoa I ··· 65

Practice 7　Protozoa II ·· 78

Practice 8　Medical arthropods ··· 92

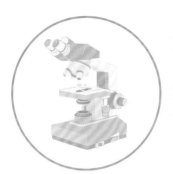

Laboratory Rules

1. Be respectful, follow teacher's instructions, and never take shortcuts.

2. Strictly adhere to all laboratory rules and regulations. Maintain a quiet environment and prioritize hygiene in the laboratory.

3. **Lab coats** must be worn upon entering the lab.

4. Remember to **bring textbook, experimental record book, and writing implements (pen/pencil/ color pencil) for graph illustrations.**

5. Follow the guidelines provided by teachers and technical staffs, and conduct experiment according to the given operating instructions. Students must obtain teacher's permission before using any instruments. Any unrelated instruments are strictly prohibited to use. Students who fail to follow the instructions and cause damage to instruments or equipment will be held responsible for the cost of repair as per university regulations.

6. Show respect and considerate treatment towards animals. Handle experimental animals with care, and wash your hands afterwards.

7. Maintain awareness of water and power safety, as well as the operational procedures of experiment materials during the course of experiment. In the event of an accident, immediately switch off the power and report to the teachers.

8. Clean the equipment and instruments after experiments and properly store them back in place. **Clean your work area and ensure it is tidy before leaving!**

9. After each experiment, students are required to write an experimental report and submit it to the teacher or the online platform of the course.

10. Eating and drinking are strictly prohibited in the lab at any time! Remain with and work within your assigned seat or group. Only leave your group or work area when instructed by the teacher. Sitting on counters or tables is not allowed.

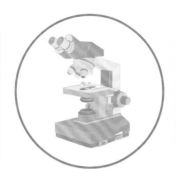

Guide for Microscope User

1. Microscopes are precise instruments composed of three main parts: a base, an arm, and a head, with additional components for illuminating, magnifying and adjustment, as depicted in **Figure 0-1.**

2. **Moving the Microscope:** Moving the microscope with two hands - one under the base and the other grasping its arm. Maintain close proximity to your body while carrying it. Careless drops are the primary cause of microscopes damage, rather than natural wear or tear.

3. **Microscope Lens Care:** Avoid touching any lens with your fingers, as this leaves oil and particles that can be hard to clean and may damage the lens. When cleaning a lens, gently wipe it with lens tissue or lens cloth. Do not use facial tissue, paper napkin, your shirt or a towel.

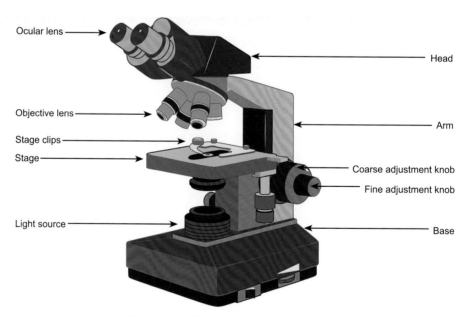

Figure 0-1　Structure of light microscope

4. **Slide Insertion:** Place the slide on the stage of the microscope, and secure it with the stage clips. For specimen requiring oil immersion, apply one drop of oil on the slide.

5. Viewing Objects

Step 1: Begin by using the lowest power objective lens to examine the samples. View the objective lens and the stage from the side, and slowly turn the coarse focus knob to move the objective lens downward. Adjust it as close to the slide as possible but avoid touching the slide.

Step 2: Look through the eyepiece and adjust the illuminator and diaphragm for optimal lighting. If you wear glasses, remove them. if you see only eyelashes, move closer and proceed.

Step 3: Slowly turn the coarse knob to raise the objective lens. Continue observing until the image becomes clear. Use fine knob for fine focusing. Once you have a clear image with the lowest power objective, you can switch to higher power objectives. You may need to readjust the sample's focus, condenser and light intensity. If you are unable to focus on the specimen, repeat steps 1 through 3 with a higher power objective lens. **Avoid contact between the objective lens and the slide!**

6. Generally, low power is suitable to view the structures of helminthic adults and larvae, while high power is better for observing eggs. Protozoa specimens commonly require an oil-immersion lens.

7. Upon completing the experiment, lower the microscope stage, switch the low power lens into the observing position, and remove the slide. Remember to clean the oil lens with lens tissue moistened with alcohol. If the specimens on the slide are not covered by a cover glass, avoid wiping the remaining oil with lens tissue to prevent damage of the specimen. Instead, gently cover the oil with lens tissue, drop alcohol on it, and carefully tear the tissure off. Repeat this process 2-3 times to ensure a complete removal of the oil.

Notes

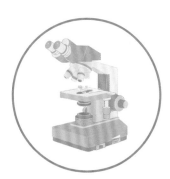

Practice 1　Nematode I

Classification

Ascaris lumbricoides (似蚓蛔线虫，蛔虫)

Hookworm:

　Ancylostoma duodenale (十二指肠钩口线虫，十二指肠钩虫)

　Necator americanus (美洲板口线虫，美洲钩虫)

Whipworm: *Trichuris trichiura* (毛首鞭形线虫，鞭虫)

Pinworm: *Enterobius vermicularis* (蠕形住肠线虫，蛲虫)

◎ Objectives

1. Identify the eggs of *A. lumbricoides*, hookworms, *T. trichiura*, and *E. vermicularis*.

2. Distinguish the adults between the two species of hookworms: *A. duodenale* and *N. americanus*.

3. Describe the morphological characteristics of adult *E. vermicularis*.

4. Differentiate the buccal capsules and the bursas between the two species of hookworms.

5. Observe the adult *A. lumbricoides* and *T. trichiura* (♀ and ♂).

Observations

(Note: Pay attention to the size, color, shape, contents of the egg, and characteristics of the shell)

1. Eggs of soil-borne nematode

(1) Eggs of *A. lumbricoides*

Two types of eggs are discharged by the adult female worms: fertilized and unfertilized eggs.

1) Fertilized eggs (Figure 1-1)

The fertilized eggs, produce after mating with the male, undergo embryonation and develop into infective eggs .

— Round or oval in shape.

— They measure (45-75) μm × (35-50) μm in size.

— Golden brown in color due to bile staining.

— The eggs have a thick, smooth, translucent shell with an outer coarsely mamillated albuminous coat, a thick transparent middle layer and an inner lipoidal vitelline membrane.

— Some eggs found in feces without the outer mamillated coat are referred to as decorticated eggs (Figure 1-2) .

— Inside the center of the egg presents a large unsegmented ovum, containing a mass of coarse lecithin granules. It occupies most of the egg, except for a clear crescentic area at each pole.

— The eggs can float on saturated salt solution.

Notes

Key point

受精蛔虫卵呈宽椭圆形，卵壳厚而透明，为所有蠕虫卵中最厚者，壳外附有一层棕黄色波浪式蛋白质膜，为子宫分泌物，从粪便排出的虫卵常被胆汁染成黄色或棕褐色。蛋白质膜如有脱落，卵壳可显示为浅黄色或无色。卵内为一未分裂的大而圆的卵细胞，卵壳与卵细胞之间多形成新月形的间隙。

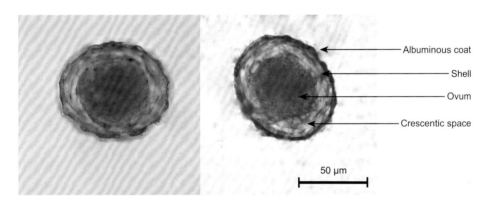

Figure 1-1　Fertilized eggs of *A. lumbricoides*

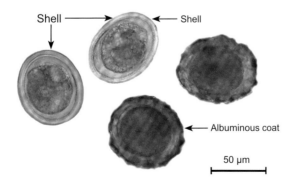

Figure 1-2　Two decorticated (top left) and two corticated (bottom right) eggs of *A. lumbricoides*

Notes

2) Unfertilized eggs

The unfertilized eggs are laid by uninseminated female. These eggs are non-embryonated and incapable of becoming infective (Figure 1-3) .

— Elliptical in shape.

— Narrower and longer than the fertilized eggs.

— Approximately (88-94) μm × (39-44) μm in size.

— These eggs have a thinner shell with irregular coating of albumin.

— Inside, they contain a small atrophied ovum accompanied by a mass of disorganized highly refractile granules of various size.

Key point

　　未受精蛔虫卵外形变化较大，常为长圆形或窄椭圆形，与受精蛔虫卵相比，卵壳和蛋白质膜均较薄，无蛔甙层，卵内充满着大小不一的折光颗粒。

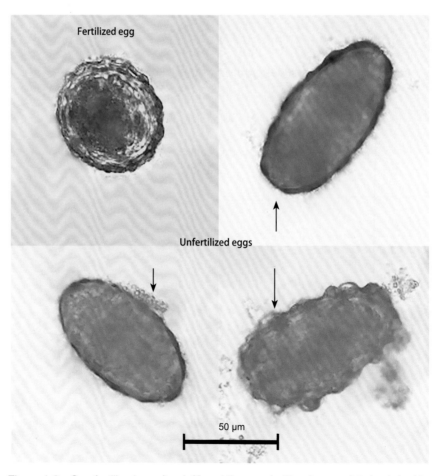

Figure 1-3　One fertilized egg (top left) and three unfertilized eggs of *A. lumbricoides*

(2) Eggs of hookworm (Figure 1-4)

— Oval or elliptical, measuring 60 μm by 40 μm.

— Colorless and are not bile-stained.

— The eggs are enveloped by a thin transparent hyaline shell membrane.

— When released by the worm in the intestine, the eggs contain an unsegmented ovum. As they passage down the intestine, the ovum undergoes development. When passed in feces, the eggs usually contain a segmented ovum with 4 or 8 blastomeres.

— A clear space can be observed between the segmented ovum and the egg shell.

— The eggs can float on saturated salt solution.

— The eggs of *A. duodenale* and *N. americanus* are similar in size and not easily distinguishable.

Notes

Key point

两种钩虫卵形态相似，难以区分，虫卵中等大小，高倍镜下呈椭圆形，两端较圆，卵壳薄，无色透明，呈细线状。卵内可见2～8个颜色不透光的卵细胞。若患者便秘或粪便放置过久，卵细胞可继续分裂为多细胞期，有时可见桑椹期甚至含蚴卵。卵壳与细胞之间有明显的间隙。

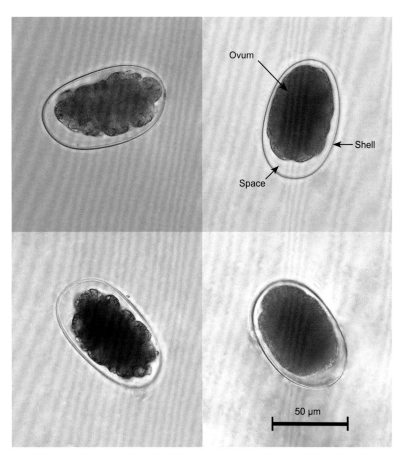

Figure 1-4   Eggs of hookworm

(3) Eggs of whipworm (Figure 1-5)

— The eggs appear brown in color and are bile-stained.

— They feature a triple shell structure, with the outermost layer being stained brown.

— The eggs have a barrel-shaped form, measuring about 50 μm in length and 22 μm in width at the middle. They exhibit a projecting mucus plug at each pole, and contain an unsegmented ovum. The plugs are colorless.

— When newly passed, the eggs contain an unsegmented ovum. At this stage, they are not infective to human.

Key point

鞭虫卵较受精蛔虫卵小，呈纺锤形或腰鼓形，黄褐色，卵壳较厚，卵壳两端各有一个透明的突起，称为盖塞或透明栓，从粪便排出的新鲜虫卵内含有一个未发育的受精卵细胞。

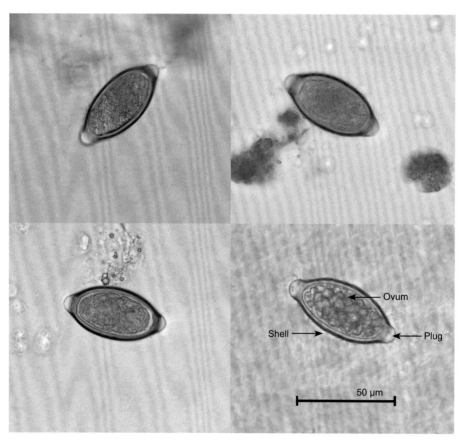

Figure 1-5　Eggs of whipworm

(4) Eggs of pinworm (Figure 1-6)

— The eggs exhibit a characteristic shape, being elongated ovoid, with one side flattened and the other convex (planoconvex) . They measure 50-60 μm by 20-30 μm.

— The egg shells are composed two layers, relatively thick, and transparent.

— Inside the eggs they contain a tadpole-shaped, coiled embryo that is fully formed. However, they become infectious quickly, around 6 hours after being deposited. If they stay in cool and moist conditions, the eggs can remain viable for approximately 2 weeks.

Notes

Key point

蛲虫卵呈长圆形，形似拉长的英文字母"D"，较受精蛔虫卵小，无色透明，两侧不对称，一侧较平，一侧稍凸，卵壳较厚。虫卵自子宫逸出时，卵细胞已发育为蝌蚪期幼虫。

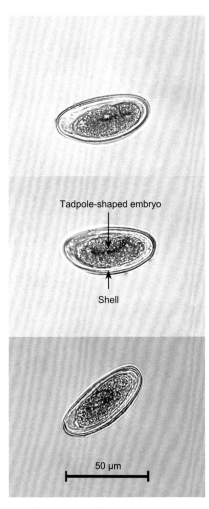

Figure 1-6   Eggs of pinworm

2. Major structures of soil-borne nematode

(1) The specific structures in the adult pinworm

— The mouth is encircled by 2 wing-like cuticular expansions known as cephalic alae (头翼), which exhibit transverse striations (Figure 1-7).

— The esophagus displays a distinctive double-bulb structure, which is a unique feature of this worm (Figure 1-8).

Key point

蛲虫成虫的鉴别要点包括在低倍镜下观察到虫体头部两端的透明延展物——头翼和食道，末端明显膨大的球形结构——食道球。这些结构有助于虫体附着于宿主肠黏膜上。

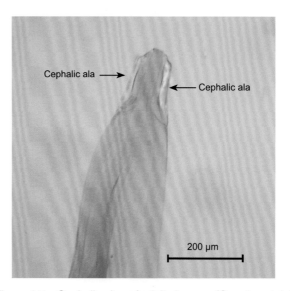

Figure 1-7　Cephalic alae of adult pinworm (Carmine stain)

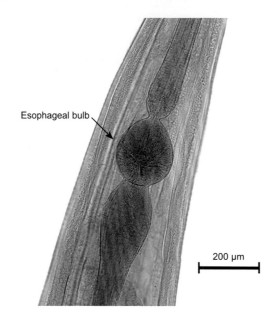

Figure 1-8　Esophageal bulb structure of adult pinworm

(Carmine stain)

Notes

(2) The buccal capsule of hookworm

The buccal capsule of *N. americanus* is characterized by a pair of cutting plates (板齿) ventrally, and 2 knob-like teeth with a median cleft dorsally. In contrast, the buccal capsule of *A. duodenale* features 4 hook-like teeth (钩齿) ventrally and 2 knob-like teeth on the dorsal surface (Figure 1-9, Figure 1-10).

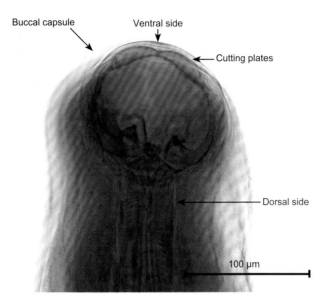

Figure 1-9　Buccal capsule of *N. americanus* (Carmine stain)

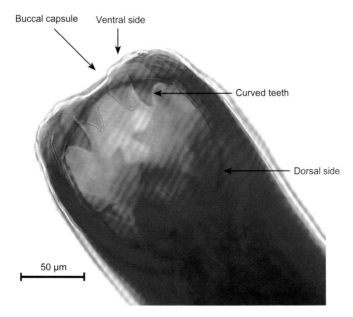

Figure 1-10　Buccal capsule of *A. duodenale* (Carmine stain)

(3) The copulatory bursa of male hookworm

Male hookworm possesses a prominent umbrella-like structure located at the posterior end, known as the copulatory bursa, which aids in copulation. The copulatory bursa is composed of 2 lateral lobes and 1 dorsal lobe. These lobes are supported by fleshy chitinous rays, which may be divided at the tip, particularly in the case of the dorsal rays. The pattern of division in the dorsal rays is useful for species differentiation. In *N. americanus,* the dorsal ray bifurcates into 2 small rays near the base of the dorsal lobe, and each small ray further separates into 2 tiny branches at the tip. On the other hand, the dorsal lobe of *A. duodenale* consists of one dorsal and two extra dorsal rays. The dorsal ray undergoes bifurcation at the tip, and each division is tripartite. (Figure 1-11, Figure 1-12) .

Key point

美洲钩虫的交合伞略扁似扇形，背幅肋由基部分为2支，每支末端又分为2小支。

十二指肠钩虫的交合伞略呈圆形，背幅肋由末端分为2支，每支末端又分为3小支。

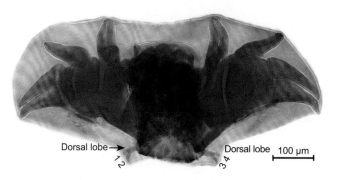

Number 1-4 indicate the branches of the dorsal rays

Figure 1-11　Copulatory bursa of *N. americanus*

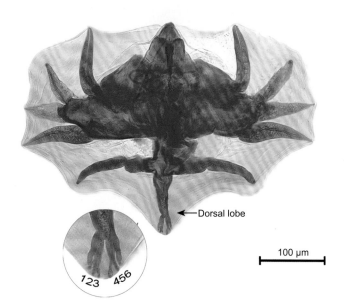

Number 1-6 indicate the branches of the dorsal rays

Figure 1-12　Copulatory bursa of *A. duodenale*

3. Morphological characteristics of adult worms

(1) Adult *A. lumbricoides*

Adult *A. lumbricoides* worms typically exhibit a creamy white color with a subtle pink hue. The cuticle, which covers the mature worms, displays fine striations. *Ascaris* adult worms are recognized as the largest intestinal nematodes. On average, adult males are slightly smaller than adult females, rarely exceeding 30 cm in length. Males are characterized by a slender and a prominent incurved tail. Adult females measure between 20 cm and 40 cm in length and a thickness similar to that of a pencil (Figure 1-13) .

 Notes

> **Key point**
>
> 蛔虫成虫形似蚯蚓，呈柱体状，中间稍膨大，两端逐渐变细，头端比尾端更显尖细。新鲜虫体呈淡红色，死后呈灰白色。口由三个呈"品"字形唇瓣构成，体表有横纹和两条侧线。雌虫大，尾部挺直且钝圆。雄虫较小，尾端向腹侧弯曲，在近尾端泄殖腔开口处，可见一对交合刺。

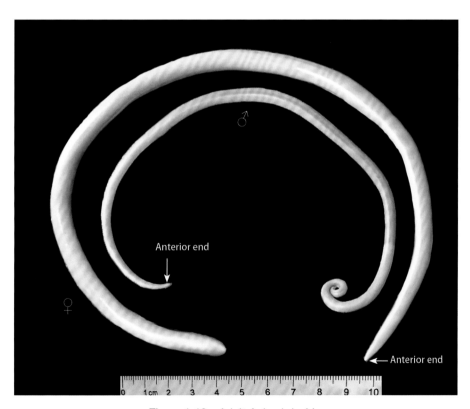

Figure 1-13   Adult *A. lumbricoides*

(2) Adult hookworms

Small adult hookworms appear grayish-white in color and possess a thick cuticle. The average adult female hookworm usually measures about 9 to 13 mm in length and 0.4 to 0.6 mm in width. Male hookworms are typically smaller, ranging from 7 to 11 mm by 0.3 to 0.5 mm in size. *N. americanus* adult is generally smaller than *A. duodenale*. The anterior end of hookworms typically forms a conspicuous bend, referred to as a hook, which gives them their name. Both *N. americanus* and *A. duodenale* have dorsally bent anterior end that features a large buccal capsule. However, the directions of these bends differ between the two species. The bend keeps the same direction along the body to the posterior end in *A. duodenale*, in contrast, the bend immediately turns into the ventral direction of the body and keeps it all the way down to the end in *N. americanus*. The hook shape is more prominent in *N. americanus* adult compared to *A. duodenale* and can serve as a distinguishing characteristic for trained observers. The posterior end of the male expands into a copulatory bursa (Figure 1-14) .

> **Key point**
>
> 钩虫成虫虫体小，呈乳白或米黄色，雌大雄小，但均约1cm。雌虫尾端钝圆，雄虫尾端膨大形成交合伞。十二指肠钩虫通体向背侧弯曲呈"C"形，美洲钩虫最前端向背侧弯曲，中部和尾端腹侧弯曲，虫体呈"S"形。

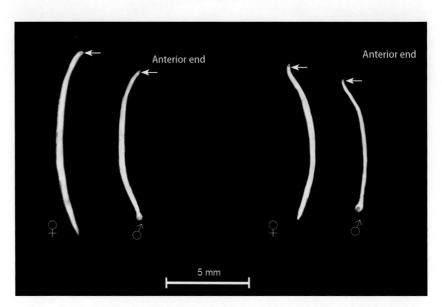

Figure 1-14　Adult hookworms，*A. duodenale* (left) and *N. americanus* (right)

(3) Adult whipworm

The typical adult whipworm measures 2.5 to 5.0 cm in length. The anterior end of the adult *T. trichiura* is significantly smaller and has a whip-like appearance, while the posterior end is larger, resembling a whip handle. These two morphologic features serve as the basis for the name whipworm. The anterior end of the adult appears colorless and contains a slender esophagus. The posterior end exhibits a pinkish-gray color, housing the intestine and reproductive systems. Adult males are generally smaller than adult females and can easily be identified by their curled tail (Figure 1-15).

Notes

Key point

鞭虫成虫形似马鞭，呈灰白色，前3/5处细长，后2/5处较粗。雌虫大，长35～50mm，尾端无弯曲；雄虫小，长30～45mm，尾端向腹面卷曲形成盘曲。

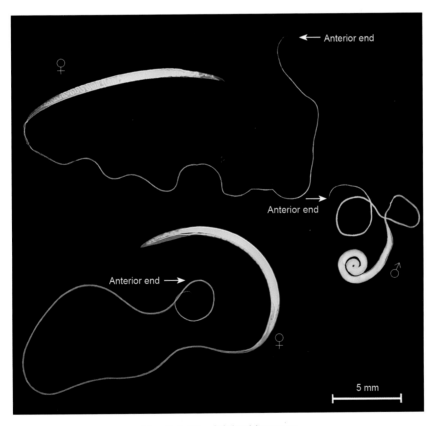

Figure 1-15   **Adult whipworms**

(4) Adult pinworm

The adult female *E. vermicularis* worm measures 7 to 14 mm in length and up to 0.5 mm in width. The yellowish-white females possess primitive organ systems, including a digestive tract, intestinal tract, and reproductive structures. In addition, the adult female exhibits a distinct clear and pointed tail that resembles a pinhead, which accounts for their common name "pinworm". The adult male worms, although rarely observed, also share a yellowish-white coloration and are typically smaller in size compared to the females, ranging from 2 to 4 mm in length and no more than 0.3 mm wide (Figure 1-16) .

> **Key point**
>
> 蛲虫成虫细小，白色，形似白色线头。雌虫长 7 ～ 14mm，虫体后 1/3 部分长而尖细；雄虫仅长 2 ～ 4mm，虫体尾端向腹面弯曲。

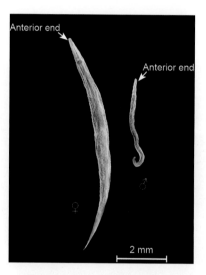

Figure 1-16　Adult pinworms

Demonstrations on the display bench

The transverse section of female *A. lumbricoides* adult (Figure 1-17)

A transverse section through a female worm reveals the characteristic structure of the body wall, consisting three layers: the outer cuticle, the hypodermis, and the somatic muscular layer on the inner side. Notably, a lateral chord projects into the pseudo-coelom and appears to have a fibrous matrix. A lateral excretory canal is embedded in the chord. The body cavity is a pseudocoel, in which all the viscera are suspended and free to move. The intestine is lined with a single layer of columnar cells. The female *A. lumbricoides* has two parallel tracts of female reproductive organs, including an ovary, oviduct, and uterus within a single tract, whereas males only possess a single tubular reproductive system.

Key point

　　以蛔虫雌虫为例，注意观察表皮及肌肉、假体腔、消化道及生殖器官。表皮为角皮层，其下为皮下层和纵肌层，皮下层伸入原体腔内并增厚，背腹及两侧分别形成4条纵索。蛔虫的表皮厚，皮下层薄，再下有肌肉层，肌细胞横截面大小不等，接近表皮的一侧较窄，伸向假体腔的肌细胞靠近体腔的一侧截面逐渐变大。消化道为狭长管状，由单层柱状上皮细胞组成，细胞的管腔面有绒毛。雌虫假体腔内可见多个卵巢、输卵管、子宫的截面。卵巢横切，可见卵原细胞为楔形，呈放射状环形排列。输卵管内有不规则空腔，呈车轮状。子宫宽大，内有虫卵截面。

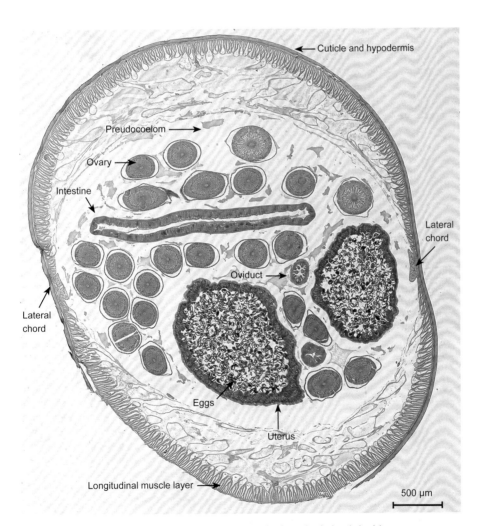

Figure 1-17　Transverse section of a female *A. lumbricoides*

Practices

Draw both fertilized and unfertilized eggs of *A. lumbricoides*, as well as the eggs of hookworm, whipworm and pinworm.

(Note: Use a pencil for drawing, sketching the outline with points and smooth lines. Avoid shading and colors. Pay attention to the accurate scales of size and shape, highlighting specific characteristics. Label the main structures accordingly.)

Quiz

1. Which of the following is the egg of *A. lumbricoides*?

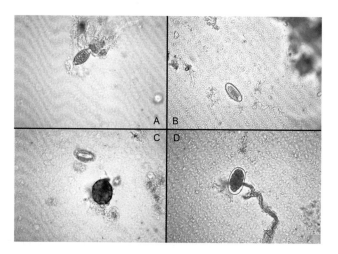

2. Which of the following is the buccal capsule of *A. duodenale*?

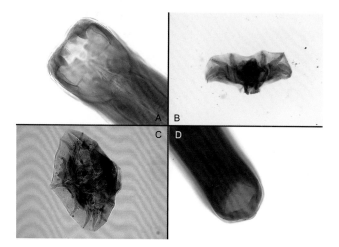

3. Differentiate between fertilized and unfertilized eggs of *A. lumbricoides*.

4. List the parasites causing autoinfection and briefly describe the life cycle of *E. vermicularis*.

5. Name the helminths that do not require an intermediate host and briefly describe the life cycle of *A. duodenale*.

Case analysis

Case 1

A survey was conducted to determine the prevalence of geohelminth infections among school-age children in China. Stool samples were collected and preserved in 10% formalin for wet mount inspection. What was observed in one of the specimens is shown in the photographs below (Figure 1-18) . The photos were taken at a magnification of 400×. What has been identified? How can this be identified?

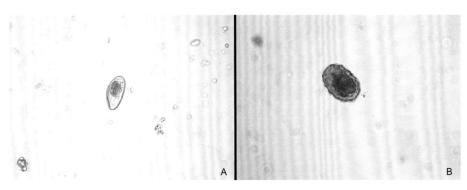

Figure 1-18   Typical objects found in the stool sample

Case 2

A 75-year-old man was referred to a local hospital due to unexplained anemia. The patient did not report any gastrointestinal complaints. During an endoscopic examination, three small worms measuring approximately 7 to 8 mm in length were found in the duodenum. The worms were observed freely in the intestinal lumen. Subsequently, the worms were taken to the parasitological department, where they were stained and mounted on slides for identification (Figure 1-19) . What is your diagnosis based on these findings?

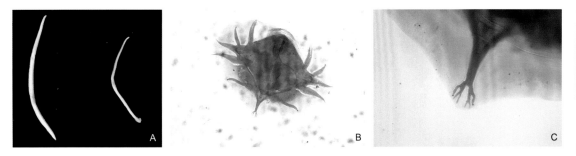

Figure 1-19   Gross (A) and microscopic(B and C) observations of the worms

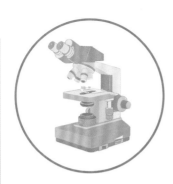

Practice 2　Namatode II

Classification

Trichinella spiralis（旋毛虫）

Filaria（丝虫）

　Brugia malayi（马来布鲁线虫，马来丝虫）

　Wuchereria bancrofti（班氏吴策线虫，班氏丝虫）

◎ Objectives

1. Describe the morphological characteristics of *T. spiralis* cysts.

2. Differentiate the morphological features between two species of microfilariae.

3. Explain the examination procedure for the encysted larvae of *T. spiralis*.

Observations

1. Stained encysted larvae (pressed muscle sample)

— Generally, 1-2 larvae (occasionally up to 6-7 larvae or more) coil up and become encysted within muscle fibers. The average size of juvenile encysted larvae ranges from 75 to 120 μm in length and 4 to 7 μm in width, with the cyst exhibiting a spindle shape (Figure 2-1).

— A fully developed larva can grow up to 1 mm in length. The longitudinal axis of the cyst generally aligns to the muscle fibers. The cyst contains a thick inner layer containing homogeneous materials derived from degraded fibroblast cells and proliferated connective tissue, as well as a thin outer layer displayed with inflammatory infiltrates.

— Biopsies of these larvae often reveal a distinctive inflammatory infiltrate in response to their presence. A striated muscle cell, known as a nurse cell, surrounds the coiled larva (Figure 2-2).

Key point

　　寄生在宿主横纹肌细胞内的幼虫卷曲于梭形囊包中，其纵轴与肌纤维走向平行。囊包内通常含 1 ～ 2 条幼虫。囊包壁由内、外两层构成，内层厚而外层较薄，内层由成肌细胞退变及结缔组织增生形成，外层可见炎症细胞浸润。

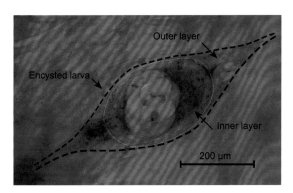

Figure 2-1   Encysted larvae (Carmine stain)

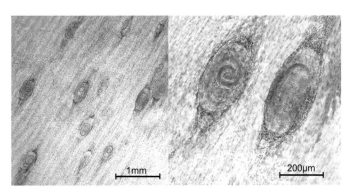

Figure 2-2   Encysted larvae in striated muscle (Iron-hematoxylin stain)

2. Microfilariae (blood smear) (Figure 2-3, Figure 2-4)

— The average microfilaria measures 240 to 300 μm in length, with a diameter of 6 to 10 μm.

— The organism is enveloped within a thin and delicate sheath.

— Numerous nuclei are present within the body.

— The cephalic or anterior end is blunt and round, featuring a distinct cephalic space devoid of nuclei.

— Near the anterior end, there is a nerve ring, followed by an excretory pore at some distance. The posterior end contains an anal spot. These structures are generally lack of nuclei.

— In comparison to *W. bancrofti*, the microfilaria cephalic space of *B. malayi* is significantly longer. The nuclei in *B. malayi* are blurred, overlapped and unequal in size, making counting difficult. In contrast, the nuclei of *W. bancrofti* microfilaria are round in shape, equal in size and scattered thus countable.

— Two discrete nuclei can be observed at the tail end of the microfilaria of *B. malayi*: one at the extreme tip of the tail and the other followed the nuclei in the body at some distance and located midway before the one at the tip. In contrast, the posterior or tail end of *W. bancrofti* microfilaria tapers to a point without nuclei.

— These key characteristics aid in distinguishing them from other sheathed microfilaria.

Key point

注意丝虫微丝蚴虫体外形、体态、鞘膜、头间隙的长宽比例、体核特征等，注意马来丝虫微丝蚴有2个尾核。

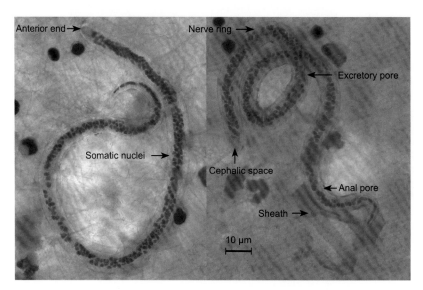

Figure 2-3　Microfilariae of *W. bancrofti* (Giemsa stain)

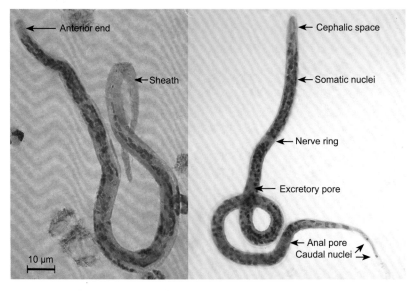

Figure 2-4　Microfilariae of *B. malayi* (Giemsa stain)

Notes

3. Adult T. *spiralis* (♀ ♂) (Figure 2-5)

These worms are thread-like and relatively small, with a slenderer anterior compared to the posterior. Adult females measure between 3 to 4 mm in length, while adult males range from 1.4 to 1.6 mm. The pharynx(咽管) is long, occupying approximately one third to half of the worm's body length. Both male and female worms have a single reproductive tract. The male lacks a copulatory spicule but possesses a large copulatory pseudobursa or clasping papilla on each side of its posterior. In female, the vulva is located near the middle of the esophagus, and the anterior portion of the uterus contains fully developed or hatched juveniles or larva.

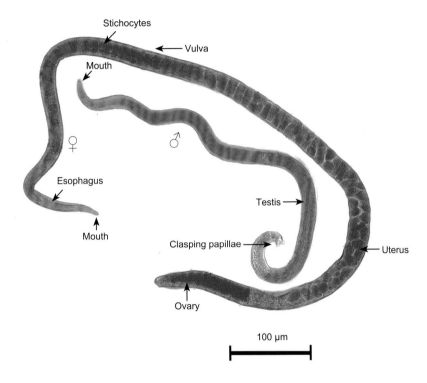

Figure 2-5   Adults of *T. spiralis* (Carmine stain)

Notes

Demonstrations on the display bench

1. Pathological section of T. *spiralis* encysted larvae in muscle tissue (Figure 2-6) .

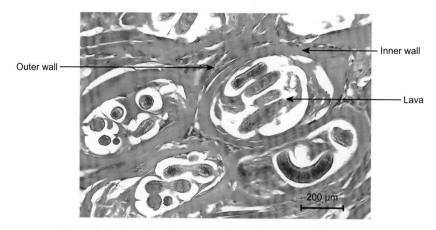

Outer wall

Inner wall

Lava

200 μm

Figure 2-6　Section of encysted larvae in muscle (H & E stain)

2. The sausage-shaped larva developed in the thoracic muscle of mosquitoes (histological tissue section) (Figure 2-7) .

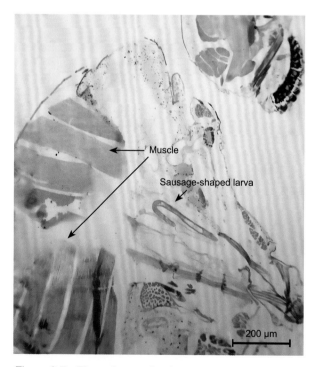

Muscle

Sausage-shaped larva

200 μm

Figure 2-7　Thoracic muscle of mosquitoes (H & E stain)

Notes

3. The releasing state of infective stage larvae (filariform larvae) from the proboscis sheath of mosquitoes (Figure 2-8) .

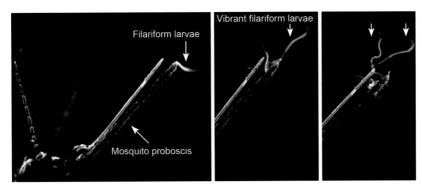

Figure 2-8   Releasing of filariform larvae from proboscis

4. Photographs depicting patients with symptoms of elephantiasis (Figure 2-9) .

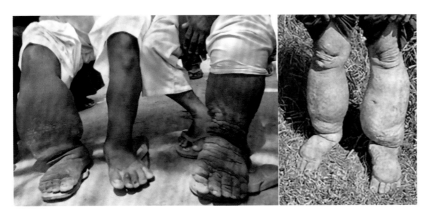

Figure 2-9   Photos of lower-limb elephantiasis

Notes

Practices

1. Draw an encysted larva.

2. Draw two species of microfilariae.

3. Outline the life cycle of *T. spiralis* using simple words and arrows.

Quiz

1. Which of the following given options is the encysted larvae of *T. spiralis*?

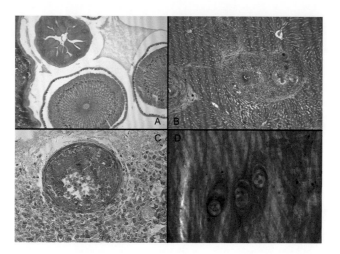

2. Which of the following given options is the microfilaria of *B. malayi* ?

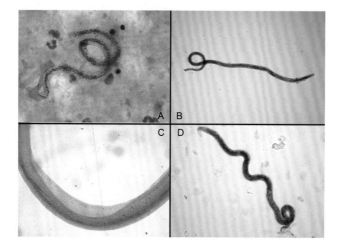

3. List various vector-borne nematodes and provide a brief description of the life cycle of silk worms.

4. Analyze why microfilariae are rarely found in the peripheral blood of patients who suffer from elephantiasis.

Case analysis

Case 1

Four construction workers presented with symptoms including stomach pain, fever, difficulty breathing, dry cough, and a skin rash. Upon investigation, it was discovered that they had recently consumed raw pork. Blood tests revealed an increase in peripheral eosinophilia. The patients provided samples of the remaining pork to the local CDC for parasitological testing. Figures show the results of compressing a small piece of meat between two slides. The images in Figure 2-10 were captured at a magnification of 200×. What is your opinion on these cases?

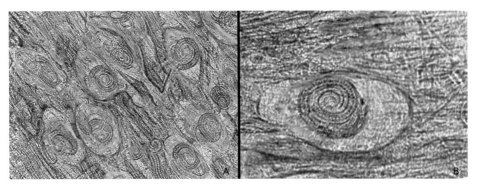

Figure 2-10　Microscopic observations of compressed meat

Case 2

Blood samples were collected from 20 individuals at a hospital for tropical diseases in coastal Indonesia, where lymphatic filariasis is endemic. Approximately one fifth of the cases were symptomatic and showed varying degrees of lymphoedema, with or without recurrent episodes of fever. The objects in Figure 2-11 were observed on Giemsa-stained thick blood films from two asymptomatic cases. These objects had an average length of 220 micrometres. What is your diagnosis? On what criteria is it based?

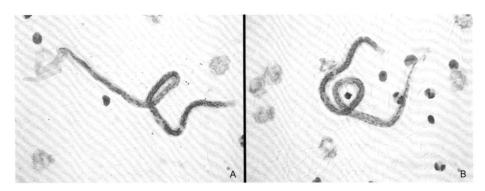

Figure 2-11　Typical observations of thick blood smear under microscope

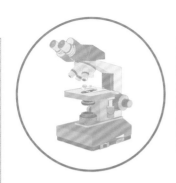

Practice 3   Trematode I

Classification

Liver fluke: *Clonorchis sinensis* (华支睾吸虫，肝吸虫)
Oriental lung fluke: *Paragonimus westermani* (卫氏并殖吸虫，肺吸虫)
Intestinal fluke: *Faciolopsis buski* (布氏姜片吸虫，肠吸虫)

◎ Objectives

Identify the eggs and adult worms of *C. sinensis*, *P. westermani*, and *F. buski*.
Describe the structures of a typical fluke adult worm, taking *C. sinensis* as an example.

Observations

1. Eggs of flukes

(1) Eggs of *C. sinensis* (Figure 3-1)

— The typical size of *C. sinensis* egg is 30 by 15 μm.

— Brown or dark brown in color.

— A developed miracidium fully occupies the interior of the egg.

— The eggs have a prominent operculum and a small knob opposite it.

— Rimmed extensions/shoulders are strategically placed around the operculum.

Key point

　　肝吸虫虫卵小，为常见虫卵中最小者，大小30 μm×15 μm，黄褐色。低倍镜下形态似芝麻，前窄后宽。高倍镜下虫卵的窄端可见一小盖，小盖与卵壳连接处增厚形成凸起的肩峰，小盖对端有一小突起称为小疣。卵随粪便被排出时，内已含有一个毛蚴。

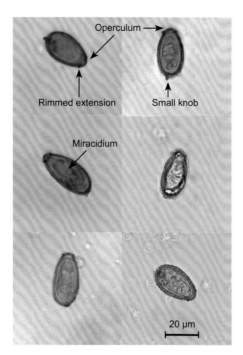

Figure 3-1   Eggs of *C. sinensis*

(2) Eggs of *P. westermani* (Figure 3-2)

— The average size of *P. westermani* eggs ranges from 80 to 118 μm in length and 48 to 60 μm in width.

— Golden yellow in color.

— The shapes are characterized by morphological variations.

— An undeveloped miracidium is enclosed in the smooth shell of the roughly round egg.

— The prominent operculum is surrounded by an opercular rim (shoulders) .

— A clear thickening can be observed within the shell, opposite the operculum.

Key point

　　肺吸虫虫卵中等大小，金黄色，呈不规则形状，多为椭圆形。虫卵一端有卵盖，大而扁平，常倾斜，有肩峰，卵壳较厚且不均匀，卵盖的对端卵壳增厚。卵内含一未发育的卵细胞和7～8个卵黄细胞。卵细胞较大而圆，折光性强。常不易观察，卵黄细胞分布不均匀，不充满整个虫卵。注意肺吸虫虫卵外形变化大，必须多看多找，掌握其特征。

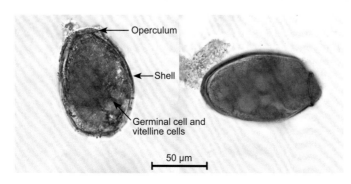

Figure 3-2   Eggs of *P. westermani*

(3) Eggs of *F. buski* (Figure 3-3)

— The size of eggs measures 130 to 140 μm by 80 to 85 μm.

— Brown in color and oblong in shape.

— With a very thin and smooth egg shell and consisting of an undeveloped ovum.

— Generally, the operculum of the eggs appears indistinct.

Key point

　　布氏姜片吸虫虫卵为人体常见寄生蠕虫虫卵中最大者，呈卵圆形，淡黄色。卵壳薄，小盖位于卵的一端，不易见，无肩峰，卵内含一未发育的卵细胞和数十个卵黄细胞。

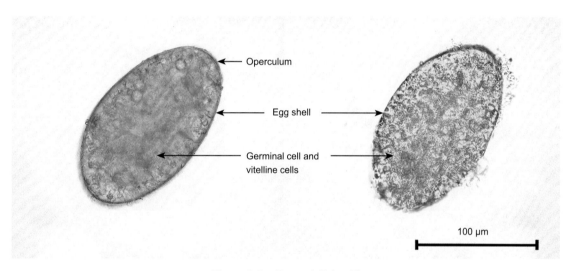

Figure 3-3　Eggs of *F. buski*

2. Adult flukes

(1) *C. sinensis* (Figure 3-4)

— The adult worm has a flat, transparent, spatulate body with a pointed anterior end and a rounded posterior end.

— It measures10 to 25 mm in length and 3 to 5 mm in width.

— The adult worm can survive in biliary tract for 15 years or more.

— The hermaphroditic worm discharges eggs into the bile duct.

Notes

Key point

　　先肉眼观察华支睾吸虫成虫玻片标本的一般形态，然后在低倍镜下观察其主要的内部结构。肉眼观察下，华支睾吸虫成虫外形呈葵花籽形。镜下可见口吸盘位于虫体最前端，腹吸盘位于虫体前1/5处，口吸盘略大。分叶状的卵巢位于虫体中与后1/3交界处，卵巢的后方有一较大的椭圆形受精囊。子宫位于虫体中1/3，迂曲盘绕，最终开口于腹吸盘前方的雌性生殖孔。卵黄腺位于虫体中部，肠管外侧自腹吸盘延伸至受精囊。2个睾丸呈分支状前后排列，约占体长的1/3。

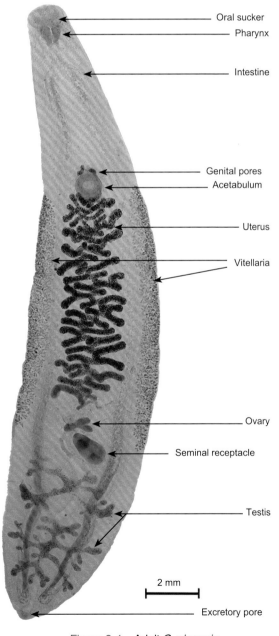

Figure 3-4　Adult *C. sinensis*

(2) *P. westermani* (Figure 3-5)

— The adult worm is egg-shaped, approximately 12 mm long, 6 mm broad, and 4 mm thick. It has a reddish brown color.

— The integument of the worm is covered with scale-like spines.

— It has an oral sucker situated anteriorly and a ventral sucker located towards the middle of the body.

— It has 2 unbranched intestinal caeca that end blindly in the caudal area.

> **Key point**
>
> 　　肉眼可见卫氏并殖吸虫形态呈宽椭圆形。口、腹吸盘大小相当，肠支粗大呈波浪状位于虫体两侧。卵巢与子宫并列于腹吸盘之后。2个睾丸位于虫体后1/3，且左右并列，卵黄腺发达，位于虫体两侧。

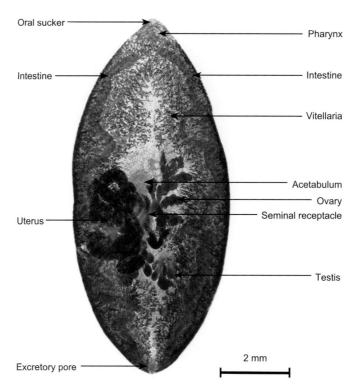

Figure 3-5　Adult *P. westermani*

(3) *F. buski* (Figure 3-6)

— The adult worm is a large, fleshy worm, measuring 20-75 mm in length, 8-20 mm in width, and 0.5-3.0 mm in thickness. It is the largest intestinal fluke affecting humans.

— It is flattened and elongated, with an ovoid shape. It has a small oral sucker and a large funnel-shaped ventral sucker (Figure 3-7) .

— Two heavily branched testes are widely distributed in posterior two third of the body, behind the ovary.

— The ovary is fan-shaped, and situated in the middle of the body.

Key point

新鲜的布氏姜片吸虫成虫呈肉红色，较肥厚，大小差异较大。经甲醛保存的虫体呈灰白色，已被压扁固定，腹吸盘靠近口吸盘，位于虫体前端。腹吸盘呈漏斗状，为口吸盘数倍，甚至肉眼可见。子宫卵巢位于腹吸盘后侧，占据虫体前半部分，睾丸高度分支呈珊瑚状，占据虫体后半部分。卵黄腺发达，分布在虫体两侧并一直延续到虫体末端。

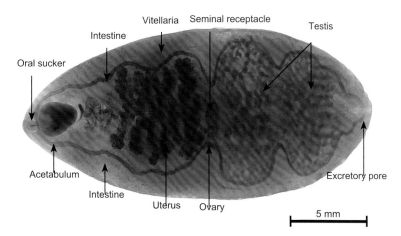

Figure 3-6　Adult *F. buski*

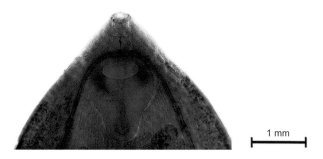

Figure 3-7　Anterior part of an adult *F. buski*

3. Histopathological section of liver flukes parasitized in hepatic bile ducts (Figure 3-8)

The transverse view of adults *Clonorchis* within a liver bile duct reveals visible structures such as the smooth tegument, muscle layers, and spongiform parenchyma. Within the parasites, the intricate structures like testes, ovaries, excretory canals, and muscular suckers may be visible. The testes are branching and blue-stained. The intestinal ceca consist of two separated tiny tubules with an epithelial lining. A section of muscular ventral/oral sucker might be present. Several egg-filled uteri can be seen close to the lobulated ovary. The biliary epithelium has significantly proliferated in the dilated bile ducts, leading to periductal fibrosis.

Key point

　　病理组织切片显示肝胆管内多个华支睾吸虫成虫的横切面。切面可能呈现吸盘、肠支、子宫、卵巢、睾丸、受精囊及卵黄腺等组织结构，不同的切面可能截取的结构不同。

　　（1）子宫：常有多个切面，宽大的子宫内可见大量虫卵。

　　（2）消化道：两个切面通常对称分布，可见上皮细胞和绒毛。

　　（3）卵巢：切面可见各级卵原细胞的核大小相差不大。

　　（4）睾丸：可有多个分支的切面，可见各级精原细胞，核的大小不一致。精子的核很小，尾部可见许多丝状结构。

　　（5）卵黄腺：位于体侧，由卵黄细胞组成，细胞内含有棕色、折光的卵黄颗粒。

　　（6）吸盘：切面可见放射状的肌肉细胞。

　　（7）体腔：各切面均未见。

　　宿主胆管上皮细胞增生，呈乳头状突向管腔，胆管周围纤维组织增生，大量炎症细胞浸润。肝细胞结构清晰，尚无明显改变。

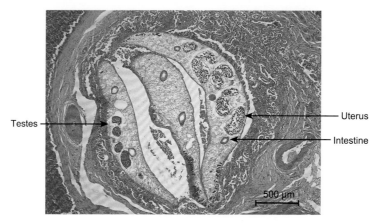

Figure 3-8　Section of liver flukes parasitized in a hepatic bile duct (H & E stain)

Demonstrations on the display bench

1. The first intermediate hosts of liver fluke are snails, such as *Parafossarulus striatulus* (纹沼螺)，*Bithynia fuchsianus* (赤豆螺)，and *Alocinma longicornis* (长角涵螺) (Figure 3-9) .

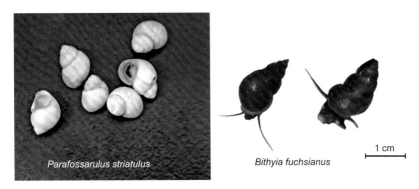

Figure 3-9   Snail hosts of liver fluke

2. The second intermediate hosts of liver fluke are fresh-water fish of the *Cyprinidae* family (Figure 3-10) .

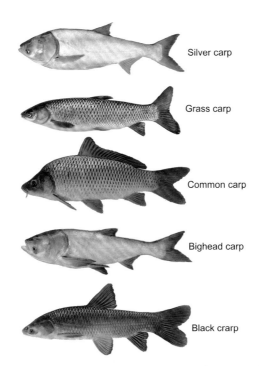

Figure 3-10   Fish hosts of liver fluke in the *Cyprinidae* family

Notes

3. The first intermediate hosts of lung fluke are in the class of *Thiaridae* and *Pleuroceridae*, with *Melania libertina* (川卷螺) being the most common species (Figure 3-11) .

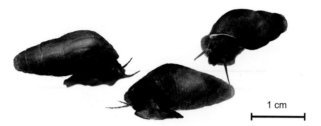

Figure 3-11　Adult *Melania libertina*

4. The second intermediate hosts of lung fluke are crabs and crayfish (Figure 3-12, Figure 3-13) .

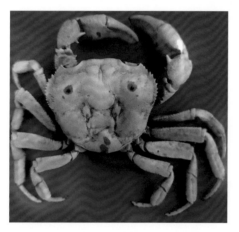

Figure 3-12　Crab host of lung fluke

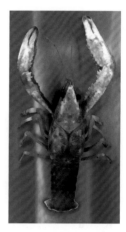

Figure 3-13　Crayfish host of lung fluke

5. The first intermediate hosts of intestinal fluke are snails of the genus *Segmentina* (扁卷螺) (Figure 3-14) .

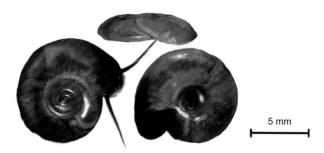

Figure 3-14　*Segmentina* host of intestinal fluke

Notes

6. Aquatic plants, such as the bulb of water chestnut（菱角）, chufa(荸荠), and roots of lotus (藕) are common vectors for transmission of *F. buski.* (Figure 3-15, Figure 3-16) .

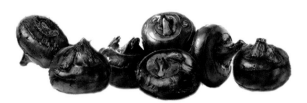

Figure 3-15   Chufa

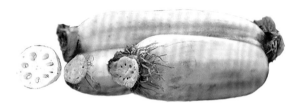

Figure 3-16   Roots of lotus

Practices

1. Draw an adult of *C. sinensis*.

2. Draw the eggs of *C. sinensis, P. westermani,* and *F. buski*.

3. Outline the life cycle of *P. westermani*.

Quiz

1. Which of the following is the egg of *C. sinensis*?

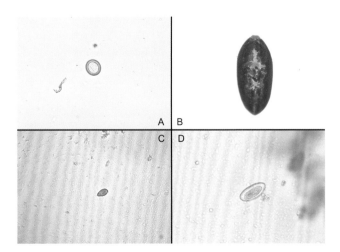

2. Which of the following is the egg of *P. westermani* ?

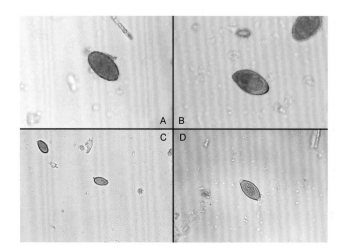

3. Which of the following is the egg of *F. buski* ?

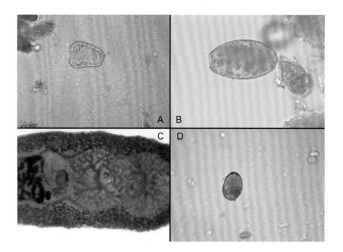

4. Describe the general characteristics of trematodes.

5. Compare the differences and similarities among the life cycles of *C. sinensis*, *P. westermani*, and *F. buski*.

Case analysis

Case 1

A young woman presented with a history of epigastric discomfort, nausea, and vomiting for a duration of 3 days. On the day of admission, the patient reported a case history of vomiting a 3-4 cm, leaf-shaped, light red worm. The worm exhibited brief movement upon expulsion and subsequently became inactive. There was no observed reduction in body weight or presence of any other constitutional symptoms. The physical examination and complete blood count (including the eosinophil count) yielded normal results. Upon further investigation, the patient provided a medical history indicating the consumption of raw vegetables washed with river water. Stool examination revealed the presence of multiple helminthic eggs observed from various perspectives (Figure 3-17 A) . Upper gastrointestinal endoscopy identified a flesh-colored plaque lesion adhering to the wall of the duodenum, measuring 2.5 cm in length and displaying an oval shape. The plaque-like lesion was successfully removed using a polypectomy snare, which exhibited noticeable twitching movement during the removal process. The worm was mounted on a slide for identification (Figure 3-17 B) . What is the diagnosis? Based on which criteria?

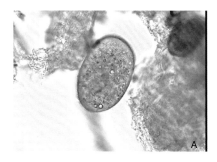
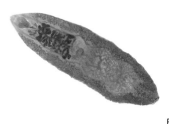

Figure 3-17   Objects in stool sample (A) and the worm (B) under microscope

Case 2

A 32-year-old Chinese man's stool sample was obtained upon his return from Thailand, where he has worked as a bridge engineer for nearly 2 years. He was asymptomatic. The stool sample was collected in 10% formalin and subjected to a formalin-ethyl acetate (FEA) concentration to carried out ova and parasites (O&P) examination. The sediment was prepared as a wet mount. The 400× magnification images in Figure 3-18 show objects measuring 25 to 30 micrometers in length. What is your opinion?

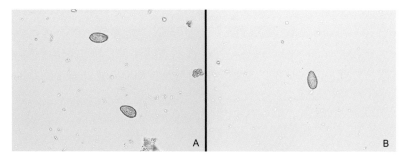

Figure 3-18   Three objects observed under microscope

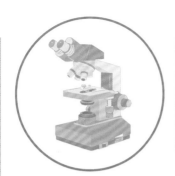

Practice 4   Trematode II

Classification

Blood fluke (血吸虫):

Schistosoma japonicum (日本血吸虫)

Schistosoma mansoni (曼氏血吸虫)

Schistosoma haematobium(埃及血吸虫)

◎ Objectives

1. Identify the eggs of *S. japonicum*.

2. Describe the morphological characteristics of miracidium, fork-tailed cercaria and adult stage of blood fluke, as well as the amphibian snails of the genus *Oncomelania*.

Observations

1. Eggs of *S. japonicum* (Figure 4-1)

— Transparent or light yellow in color, and ovoid in shape.

— Measuring 50 to 89 μm by 38 to 67 μm.

— The eggs are characterized by the presence of a small lateral spine, which can often be challenging to detect under microscopic examination.

— No operculum is found on the shell.

— Tissue debris is often found to stick around the shell due to the release of egg from the site of intestinal mucosal necrosis.

— One egg often contains a miracidium.

Key point

　　日本血吸虫虫卵比受精蛔虫卵稍大，呈宽椭圆形，淡黄色。卵壳薄厚均匀，无卵盖，壳外常附有坏死组织，壳的一端常可见一特征性的透明小棘，因虫卵的位置关系有时不可见。卵内有胚膜，胚膜内有一成熟的毛蚴，毛蚴与胚膜和卵壳之间有油滴状的代谢产物。

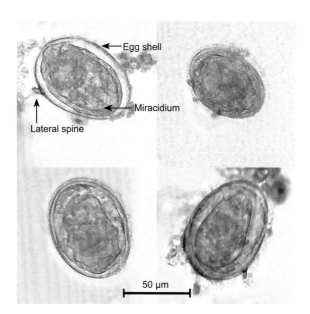

Figure 4-1   Eggs of *S. japonicum*

2. Adults of *S. japonicum* (♀ ♂) (Figure 4-2,Figure 4-3,Figure 4-4)

Blood flukes are dioecious. Both adult worms are bilaterally symmetrical and have oral and ventral suckers for attachment and stabilization. The esophagus transits into fork-shaped intestinal ceca at the level of the ventral sucker. Near the posterior end, the ceca reunite to form a blind-ended cecum. The male worm, milky-white in color, has a ventral, longitudinal groove called the gynecophoral canal (抱雌沟) , where the longer and slenderer grayish-brown female normally resides. Males measure approximately 1.5 cm by 0.5 mm and have smooth skin. Seven ellipsoid testes are aligned one behind the other, slightly posterior to the ventral sucker. Females typically measure around 2.0 cm by 0.3 mm. The ellipsoid ovary is situated near the middle of the body. The uterus extends from the middle of the body to the genital pore and may contain hundreds of eggs. The vitelline glands occupy the posterior half of the female worm.

Key point

　　日本血吸虫雌雄异体，雌雄虫均具有口、腹吸盘，腹吸盘突出体表。肠管在腹吸盘后缘水平分为左右2支，延伸到虫体中部后再汇合成单一管道到虫体末端。注意观察雄虫生殖器官的特征，包括睾丸数目、形态、位置和排列方式；雌虫卵巢、子宫、子宫内的虫卵、卵黄腺的形态特征。雄虫前端有一漏斗状的口吸盘，稍后面即腹吸盘，自腹吸盘向后，虫体逐渐扁平，并两侧卷曲为筒状，中间即为抱雌沟。睾丸呈卵圆形，一般为7个单行排列于腹吸盘的背面稍下方。雌虫虫体细长，口、腹吸盘均较雄虫小，有1个卵巢，呈椭圆形，位于虫体中央，卵黄腺排列比较规则，位于虫体后1/4的两侧，卵巢的前方为卵模，由卵模向前发出一长管状的子宫。雌虫和雄虫常合抱于抱雌沟内，雄虫较粗短呈灰白色，雌虫细长呈灰黑色。

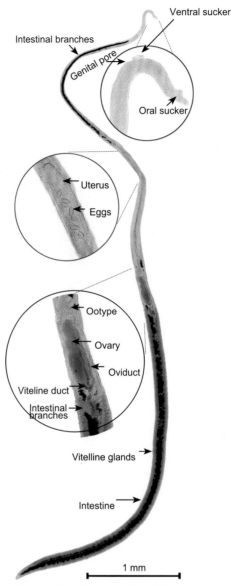

Figure 4-2   Female adult of *S. japonicum*

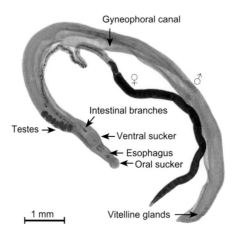

Figure 4-3   Pairing adults of *S. japonicum*

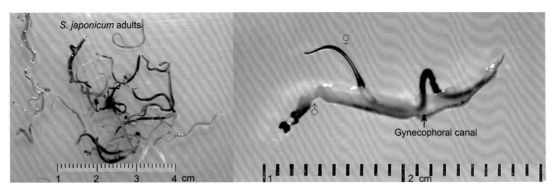

Figure 4-4 Gross specimen of adult *S. japonicum*

3. Cercaria of *S. japonicum* (Figure 4-5)

The fork-tailed cercaria measures (280-360) μm × (50-100) μm in size. It has a long tail of approximately the same size as the body, and the furci are 60-100 μm in length. The front end of cercaria is equipped with an array of glands, an oral sucker, and a ventral sucker for entering a definitive host.

Key point

日本血吸虫尾蚴为叉尾型，分体、尾两部分，体部呈长椭圆形，前端有一较大的口吸盘，其后部有一较小腹吸盘。尾部较长，其末端分叉，分叉的长度小于尾干的一半。

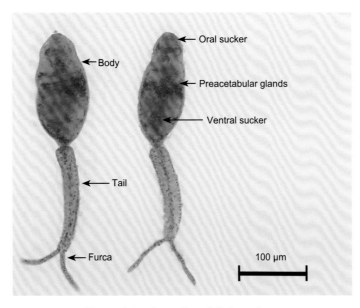

Figure 4-5 Cercariae of *S. japonicum*

4. Histopathological section of human liver with egg granuloma (Figure 4-6)

Human liver pathology reveals inflammatory infiltration centered around clustered eggs. In the portal triads, several thin-shelled eggs, some collapsed and twisted, can be observed. The black stains eggs indicate calcification. Over time, the pathological changes are generally categorized into two distinct stages: the acute phase and the chronic phase. Sections with acute stage show infiltration of eosinophils, leucocytes, and radiating acidophilic streaks surrounding fresh eggs. The sections with chronic stage commonly display dead or calcified eggs surrounded by epithelioid cells, multinucleated giant cells, and fibroblasts. High level of eosinophil infiltration is the primary characteristic of egg granuloma.

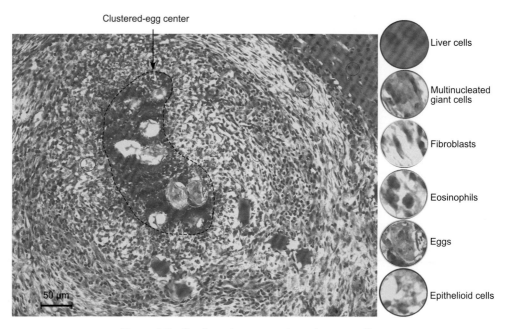

Figure 4-6　Section of egg granuloma in mouse liver

5. Eggs of *S. mansoni* (Figure 4-7)

— Measuring 114 to 175 μm by 45 to 70 μm.

— Have a transparent shell with a sharp lateral spine (侧刺) .

— When passed in feces, they contain a miracidium.

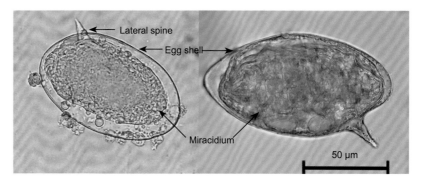

Figure 4-7　Eggs of *S. mansoni*

6. Eggs of *S. haematobium* (Figure 4-8)

— Measuring 112 to 170 μm in length and 40 to 70 μm in width
— Have a transparent shell with a sharp terminal spine (端刺).
— Containing a miracidium when voided in urine.

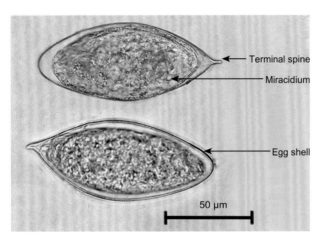

Figure 4-8   Eggs of *S. haematobium*

Demonstrations on the display bench

1. The unique intermediate host of *S. japonicum*: Snails of the genus *Oncomelania* (Figure 4-9).

Key point

肉眼观察日本血吸虫唯一中间宿主——钉螺，可见其外形呈尖塔状，侧面呈细长三角形，一般高约1cm。螺壳由螺旋围绕形成，平均为7个半圈，螺壳表面平滑的称为光壳钉螺，螺壳表面粗糙且具有凸起纵肋的称为肋壳钉螺。在壳口外唇后方有一条淡黄色紧贴外唇的肥厚隆起称为唇嵴，是钉螺与其他螺蛳相区别的特征之一。在活标本的壳口处可见透明角质的厣（音眼），附着于腹足后侧，钉螺受到扰动或环境变干燥时，厣即封闭壳口保护软体，也可防止体液损失。

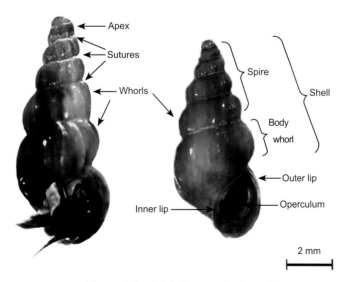

Figure 4-9   Adult *Oncomelania* snail

2. Miracidium of *S. japonicum*: The miracidium, measuring 99 × 35 μm in size, is an ovoid, ciliated, free-swimming organism with a non-functional digestive tract (Figure 4-10).

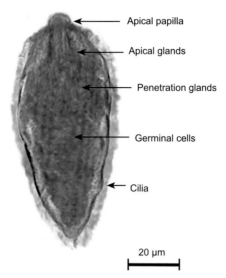

Figure 4-10   Miracidium of *S. japonicum* (Masson's stain)

Practices

1. Dissection of mouse model infected with *S. japonicum*

1) Smash a cercaria-positive snail, place it between two slides, and add a drop of water to the debris to maintain the vitality of released cercaria. Put the slides under the microscope to observe living cercariae. Be caution, direct skin exposure to cercariae may get infected.

2) Sacrifice mice at 6 weeks post-infection and examine the peritoneal cavity (Figure 4-11A). Note the pathological lesions in spleen (Figure 4-11B), liver (Figure 4-11C and E), and rectum (Figure 4-11D). Locate and isolate the adults from the portal vein and mesenteric veins. Put them under a stereoscope (体视镜) to observe their vitality and morphology.

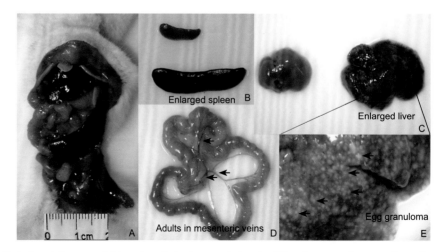

Arrows indicate the adult worms of *S.japonicum* living in mesenteric veins (D) and egg granulomas on the surface of liver (E).

Figure 4-11   Dissected mice and enlarged organs after infection

3) Take a small piece of infected liver tissue where egg granuloma can be observed, and press it between two slides for microscopic examination. Note the accumulation of the eggs resembled like grapes in the liver (Figure 4-12).

Notes

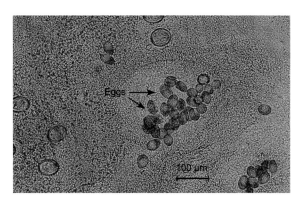

Figure 4-12   Egg granuloma in mouse liver

2. Draw a pair of adults of *S. japonicum*, highlighting the suckers, testes, ovary, intestinal tube and vitellaria.
3. Draw an egg of *S. japonicum*.
4. Outline the life cycle of *S. japonicum* using brief text and arrows.

Quiz

1. Which one is the egg of *S. japonicum*?

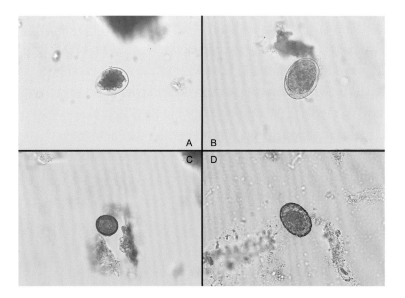

2. Which one is the female adult or the part of female adult of *S. japonicum*?

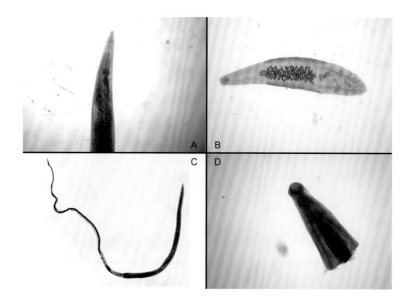

3. How many stages of *S. japonicum* can cause pathogenesis in human host, which stage is the most harmful, and why?

Case analysis

Case

A 57-year-old man who had been working in Southeast Asia for eight months returned to China and experienced symptoms such as abdominal pain, cramps, and diarrhea. Considering his travel history, a routine examination of his stool was conducted to detect O & P. The examination revealed several objects in the stool sample, as depicted in Figure 4-13. These objects were observed under a magnification of 400×. The object in Figure 4-13 A was approximately 75 micrometers long and 50 micrometers wide, presenting in large numbers. Figure 4-13 B depicts objects measuring around 60 micrometers in length and 40 micrometers in width, presenting in moderate numbers. Figure 4-13 C and D show an object measuring approximately 25 micrometers long and 15 micrometers wide, also presenting in moderate numbers.The presence of these objects in stool sample suggests a potential parasitic infection. Diagnosis would likely be confirmed by your analysis and identification.

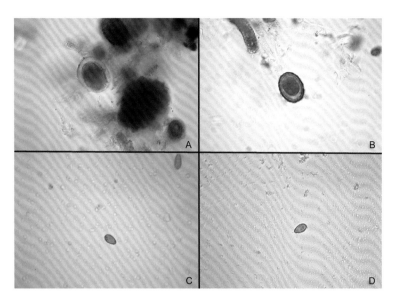

Figure 4-13   Typical objects found in stool sample

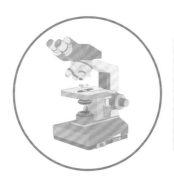

Practice 5   Cestode

Classification

Pork tapeworm: *Taenia solium* (猪带绦虫)
Beef tapeworm: *Taenia saginata* (牛带绦虫)
Hymenolepis nana (微小膜壳绦虫)
Echinococcus granulosus (细粒棘球绦虫)
Echinococcus multilocularis (多房棘球绦虫)
Spirometra mansoni (曼氏迭宫绦虫)

◎ Objectives

1. Identify and characterize the eggs of *T. solium*.

2. Describe the morphological differences between the adult worms of *T. solium* and *T. saginata*, focusing on the scolex, mature proglottids and gravid proglottids.

3. Distinguish the morphology of hydatid, hydatid sand(棘球蚴砂), and protoscolex.

Observations

1. Eggs

(1) Eggs of *T. solium* (Figure 5-1)

— The eggs of *Taenia spp.* share a similar appearance and cannot be differentiated by naked eye.

— Spherical or sub-spherical in shape.

— Measuring 31-43 μm.

— The eggshell, a thin hyaline embryonic membrane, is seldom visible after release due to its fragility.

— Each egg contains an oncosphere surrounded by a thick, radially striated embryophore (inner wall) that appears yellow-brown due to bile staining.

— In the center, the fully-developed embryo (oncosphere) can be identified by 3 pairs of hooklets (hexacanth embryo) .

Notes

（Key point）

　　10倍镜下带绦虫卵形似水中小气泡，较受精蛔虫卵小。在40倍镜下呈圆形，黄褐色，外层为胚膜，胚膜为褐色具放射状条纹，其内含六钩蚴，可见3对透明的小钩。完整虫卵外有卵壳，因其无色透明且薄而易碎，随粪便排出时带绦虫卵卵壳大多破碎脱落，实为胚膜包裹的六钩蚴。

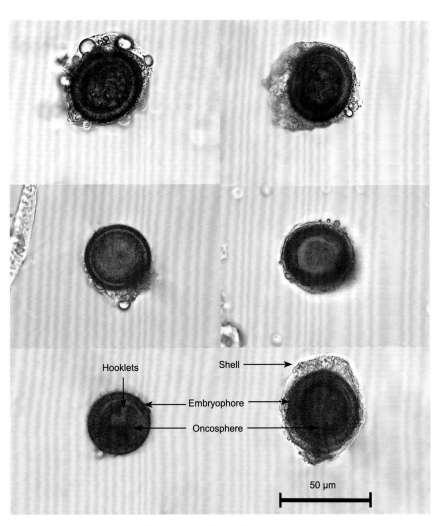

Figure 5-1　Eggs of *T. solium*

(2) Eggs of *Hymenolepis nana* (Figure 5-2)

— Roughly spherical or ovoid in shape, measuring 30-40 μm.

— They possess a thin colorless outer membrane and inner embryophore that enclosed a hexacanth oncosphere.

— The space between the two membranes contains yolk granules and 4-8 thread-like polar filaments arising from two knobs on the embryophore.

> **Key point**
>
> 微小膜壳绦虫卵呈椭圆形，无色透明，比受精蛔虫卵稍小，卵壳薄，卵内有胚膜，较厚，其两端各有一突起，并各发出4～8根丝状物，卵壳与胚膜之间充满透明而半流动的物质，胚膜内含一发育成熟的六钩蚴。

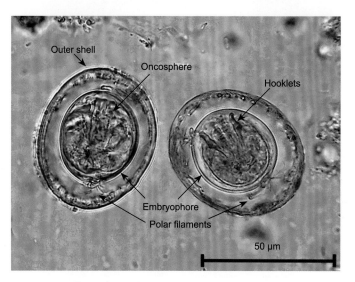

Figure 5-2　Eggs of *Hymenolepis nana*

2. Proglottid

(1) Mature proglottid

The mature proglottids of both *Taenia* species exhibit similar morphological characteristics. The testes consist of multiple follicles randomly distributed throughout. The uterus is tubular and may or may not have small branches at the blind end. In *T. saginata*, the ovary consists of only two lobes (Figure 5-3) , whereas *T. solium* has a small accessory lobe (Figure 5-4) in addition to the two main lobes. The digestive organs cannot be observed.

> **Key point**
>
> 两种带绦虫成节结构大体相同。每个节片都有雌雄生殖器官，子宫呈囊状，无子宫孔，卵巢分两叶，猪带绦虫卵巢另有一中央小叶；睾丸呈滤泡状均匀分布。

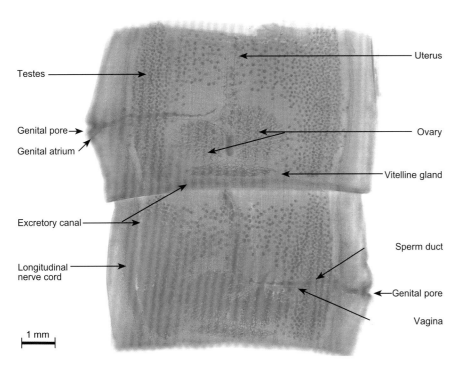

Figure 5-3   Mature proglottid of *T. saginata*

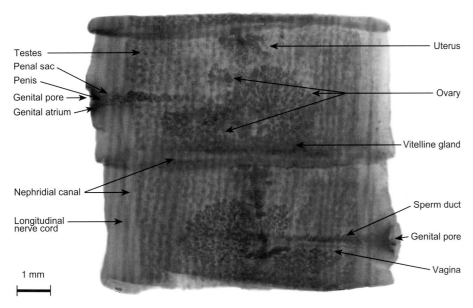

Figure 5-4   Mature proglottid of *T. solium*

(2) Gravid proglottid (ink-stained)

The mature segments of *T. saginata* are approximately four times longer than their width, measuring around 20 mm in length and 5 mm in width. The uterus is extensively branched, typically consisting of 15-30 lateral branches on each side by counting the primary branches directly from the stem of it in *T. saginata* (Figure 5-5) . In contrast, *T. solium* gravid proglottids have 7-13 lateral branches (Figure 5-6) . The number of branches is an important distinguishing factor between *Taenia* species(Table 5-1).

Key point

　　肉眼观察：猪带绦虫孕节内从子宫主干单侧基部发出的分支数量为7 ～ 13支，牛带绦虫孕节内从子宫主干单侧基部发出的分支数量为15 ～ 30支。注意只有子宫主干直接分出的分支计算在内，末端的再分支不作为计算的依据。子宫单侧的分支数是鉴别两种绦虫的重要依据。

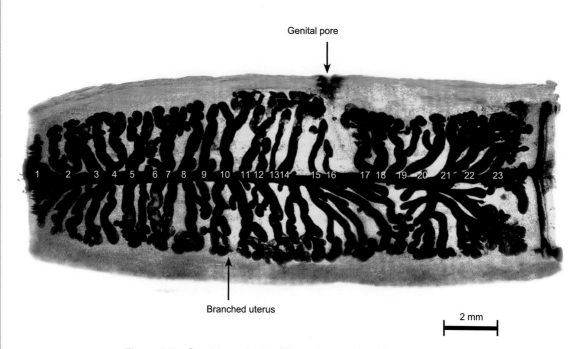

Figure 5-5　Gravid proglottid of *T. saginata* with 23-branch uterus

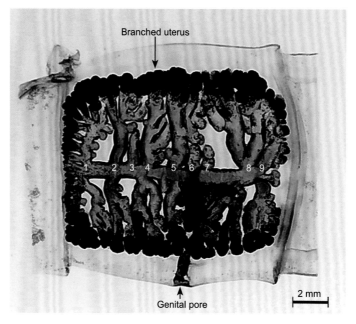

Figure 5-6　Gravid proglottid of *T. solium* with 9-branch uterus

Table 5-1   Difference between *T. saginata* and *T. solium*

	T. saginata	*T. solium*
Length	5-10 m	2-3 m
Scolex	Large quadrate	Small and globular
	Rostellum and hooks are absent	Rostellum and hooks are present
	Suckers may be pigmented	Suckers not pigmented
Neck	Long	Short
Proglottids	1 000-2 000	Below 1 000
Measurement (gravid segment)	5-20 mm	6-12 mm
Expulsion	Expelled singly	Expelled passively in chains of 5 or 6
Uterus	Lateral branches 15-30 on each side; thin and dichotomous	Lateral branches 5-10 on each side; thick and dendritic
Vagina	Present	Absent
Accessary lobe of ovary	Absent	Present
Testes	300-400 follicles	150-200 follicles
Larva	Cysticercus bovis; present in cow not in human	Cysticercus cellulosae; present in pig and also in human
Egg	Not infective to human	Infective to human
Definitive host	Human	Human
Intermediate host	Cow	Pig, occasionally human
Disease	Causes intestinal taeniasis	Causes intestinal taeniasis and cysticercosis

Notes

Demonstrations on the display bench

1. Scolex

(1) *T. solium*: small and globular, measuring approximately 1 mm in diameter. It possesses 4 large cup-like suckers (0.5 mm in diameter) and a conspicuous rounded rostellum. The rostellum is armed with a double row of hooks, numbering 20-50, which alternate between round and small dagger-shaped hooks (Carmine stain) (Figure 5-7) .

Key point

　　猪带绦虫头节染色标本呈圆球状，具有4个吸盘，顶端具有顶突，顶突上有内大外小两圈小钩，颈部紧连头节，窄细，后续链体。

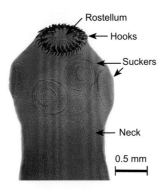

Figure 5-7　Scolex of *T. solium*

(2) *T. saginata*: 1-2 mm in diameter, and is quadrilateral in cross-section. It bears 4 hemispherical suckers situated at its four angles. Unlike *T. solium*, *T. saginata* lacks the rostellum and hooklets, earning it the name "unarmed tapeworm". The suckers serve as the sole organ for attachment (Carmine stain) (Figure 5-8) .

Key point

　　牛带绦虫头节染色标本呈近似方形，具有4个吸盘，无顶突和小钩。

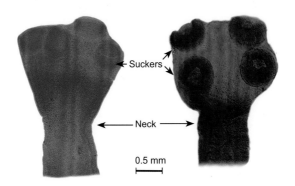

Figure 5-8　Scolex of *T. saginata*

2. Adult worm

(1) *T. solium*: The adult worm is typically 2-4 meters long and has fewer than a thousand pro-glottids. The proglottids resemble those of *T. saginata* in general (Figure 5-9) .

Key point

猪带绦虫成虫体长2～4m，乳白色，半透明，前端窄，后端宽，其未成熟节片宽大于长，成熟节片长宽相等，妊娠节片长大于宽，生殖孔呈左右不规则排列。

Notes

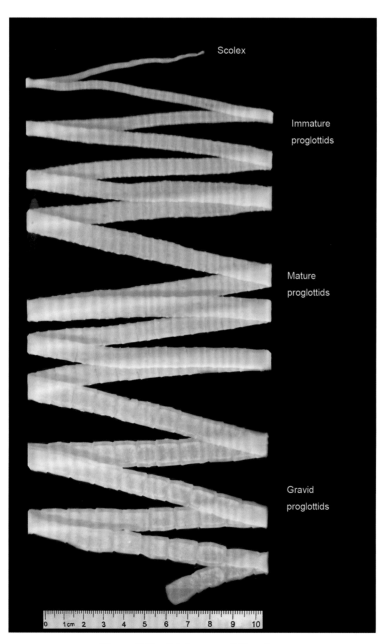

Figure 5-9　Adult worm of *T. solium*

(2) *T. saginata*: The mature *T. saginata* worm is 4-8 m in length and exhibits an opalescent white color. It has a ribbon-like, dorsoventrally flattened shape and is segmented. The worm possesses a long, thin neck, and the strobila is divided into immature, mature, and gravid proglottids (Figure 5-10) .

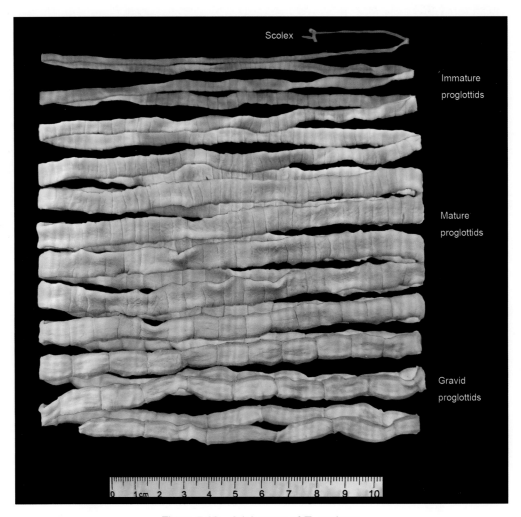

Figure 5-10   Adult worm of *T. saginata*

Notes

3. Cysticercus cellulose

The cysticercus cellulose is an opalescent milky-white ovoid structure, measuring 8-10 mm in length and 5 mm in width (Figure 5-11) .

Key point

猪囊尾蚴呈卵圆形，乳白色，半透明，囊中充满液体，其头节由囊壁内凹形成一白色圆点，形似白米粒。

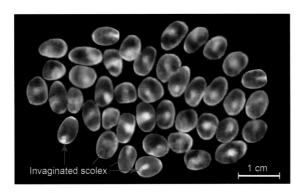

Figure 5-11   Cysticercus cellulose of *T. solium*

4. Different stages of *E. granulosus*

(1) Adult worm of *E. granulosus*: This small tapeworm measures only 3-6 mm in length and consists of a scolex, short neck, and strobila. The strobila is composed of only 3 proglottids: the anterior immature, middle mature, and posterior gravid proglottid (Figure 5-12) .

Key point

细粒棘球绦虫虫体小，通常只有4个节片，包括头节、未成熟节片、成熟节片和孕节，有时可见2个孕节。

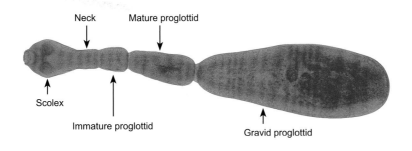

Figure 5-12   Adult worm of *E. granulosus*

(2) The eggs of *Echinococcus* cannot be distinguished from those of *Taenia* species. They are ovoid, brown in color, and contain an embryo with 3 pairs of hooklets (Figure 5-13) .

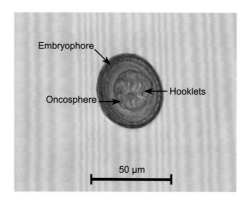

Figure 5-13　Egg of *E. granulosus*

(3) Hydatid cyst or hydatid sand: It refers to a hollow bladder or cyst filled with fluid. The diameter can range from 0.5-1.0 cm or even larger. The cyst wall, secreted by the embryo, consists of 3 indistinguishable layers: the outer pericyst, intermediate ectocyst and inner endocyst. The interior of the cyst contains clear, colorless or pale-yellow fluid (hydatid fluid) . At the bottom of cyst, there is granular deposit or hydatid, comprising free brood capsules, protoscolices and loose hooklets, just like the property of sand, so it is called "hydatid sand." (Figure 5-14) .

Key point

　　棘球蚴砂染色玻片标本内可见棘球蚴囊中所含的原头蚴和子囊等，低倍镜下头节呈圆形，其顶突和小钩由顶端凹入，染色较深呈圆形处即为吸盘所在，4个吸盘一般不易见。

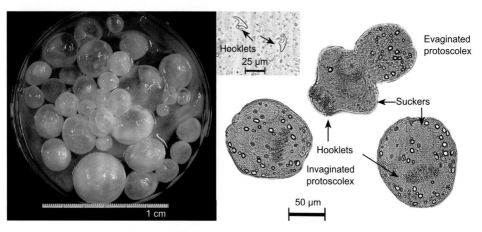

Figure 5-14　Hydatid cysts of *E. granulosus*

(4) Gross specimen of hydatid cysts: This refers to a hepatic mass of hydatid cyst resected from a hydatid patient (Figure 5-15) .

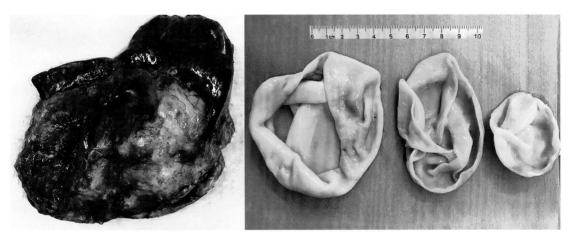

Figure 5-15   A view of resected cysts (left) and germinative membranes (right)

5. Different stages of *S. mansoni*

(1) Eggs: The eggs of Spirometra resemble those of digenetic trematode. They are oval, yellow-brown in color, and possess a distinct operculum at one pole of the shell. The average dimension of the eggs is 60 μm by 36 μm. Spirometra eggs have an asymmetric appearance and tend to be pointed at one end, with a slight bump might present on the opercular end. The eggs are unembryonated when passed in the feces. Cats may have extended periods with negative fecal samples followed by periods with present eggs excretion (Figure 5-16) .

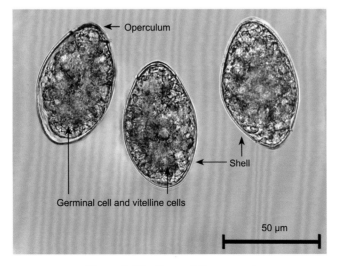

Figure 5-16   Eggs of *S. mansoni*

(2) Scolex: The scolex of *S. mansonoides* lacks suckers but instead possesses two shallow longitudinal grooves called bothria. It varies in diameter from 0.2 mm to nearly 0.5 mm, with bothria approximately 1.0 mm in length. The bothria shallow, broad, and a flat bottom (Figure 5-17).

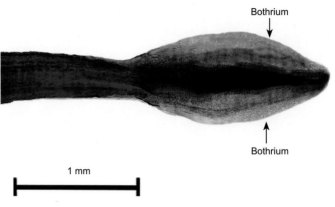

· Figure 5-17　Scolex of *S. mansoni*

(3) Sparganum: Sparganum (plerocercoid larva) of *S. mansoni* is white, wrinkled, and ribbon-shaped. It ranges in length from a few millimeters to several centimeters. The anterior end possesses sucking grooves, similar to those present in the scolex of the mature worm (Figure 5-18).

Key point

肉眼观察曼氏迭宫绦虫裂头蚴标本可见裂头蚴呈长条形，约300mm×0.7mm，体前端稍大，具有与成虫相似的头节，呈指状，在其背腹面各有一纵行的吸槽，体不分节，但具有横纹。

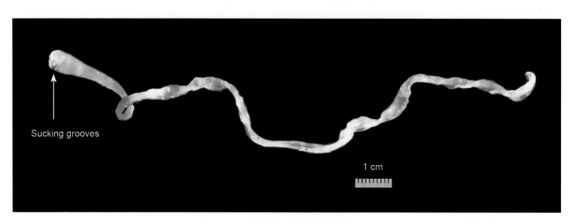

Figure 5-18　Sparganum of *S. mansoni*

Practices

1. Dissection of a mouse model infected with *E. multilocularis*

1) Please observe the mess lesions in the mouse abdomen (Figure 5-19 A).

2) Sacrifice the mice of four-month post infection and open the peritoneal cavity. Notice the numerous alveolar hydatids in various sizes (Figure 5-19 B). Observe the pathological invasions of the hydatids in the liver and the enlargement of the mouse spleen. Note that the cysts metastasize from the liver and fill the body cavity. Isolate the hydatids into a Petri dish (Figure 5-19 C).

3) Slice a piece of hydatid and press it between two slides. Examine the slides under a light microscope. Observe the protoscolices accumulated in hydatid cysts (Figure 5-19 D).

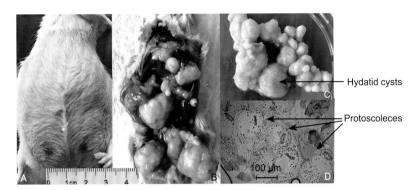

Figure 5-19   Alveolar hydatid cysts in mouse

2. Draw a *Taenia* egg and a gravid proglottid.

3. Draw scolices of *T. solium* and *T. saginata*, and provide labels for each structure.

4. Outline the life cycle of *T. solium* with concise text and arrows.

Quiz

1. Which one is the egg of *T. solium*?

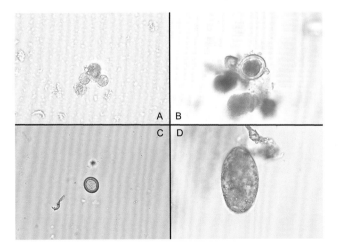

2. Which one is the gravid proglottid of *T. saginata*?

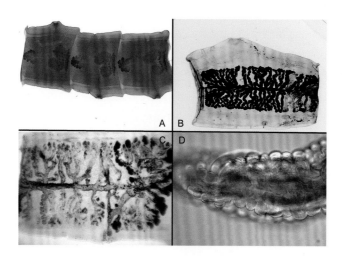

3. How to distinguish *T. solium* and *T. saginata* in terms of their morphology, life cycle, pathogenesis, and epidemical characteristic?

4. How can one determine if a tapeworm infection has been successfully treated? Why is it important to conduct a curative effect examination for tapeworm infections?

Case analysis

Case

A 25-year-old man reported observing worm-like objects in his feces. He had spent three months in India one year prior and had previously noticed white items in his stool at that time. Stool samples were collected and sent to the local hospital clinical laboratory for examination. Additionally, stool samples were collected in 10% formalin for further investigation. Figure 5-20 A shows the worm-like object following ink injection. Figure 5-20 B depicts what was found on a moist, unstained mount of stool in low numbers. The items of interest had an average dimension of 30-34 μm. What has been found? Share your opinion.

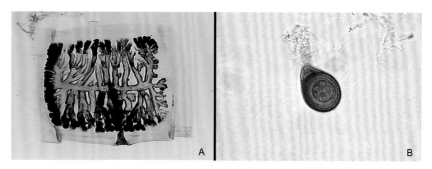

Figure 5-20　Objects found under microscope in feces (A) and stool sample (B)

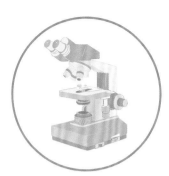

Practice 6　Protozoa I

Classification

Entamoeba histolytica (溶组织内阿米巴)

Entamoeba coli (结肠内阿米巴)

Giardia lamblia (蓝氏贾第鞭毛虫)

Trichomonas vaginalis (阴道毛滴虫)

Leishmania donovani (杜氏利什曼原虫)

◎ Objectives

1. Identify the mature cysts of *E. histolytica, E. coli,* and *G. lamblia.*

2. Distinguish the trophozoites of *E. histolytica*, *G. lamblia* and *T. vaginalis,* as well as the amastigote and promastigote of *L. donovani.*

Observations

1. Trophozoites and cysts (under oil immersion lens)

(1) Trophozoites of *E. histolytica* (Iron-hematoxylin stain) (Figure 6-1)

— The trophozoites are irregular in shape and vary in size from 10-60 μm.

— The outer ectoplasm is clear, transparent, and refractile, while the inner endoplasm is finely granular with a ground glass appearance.

— The endoplasm contains a nucleus, food vacuoles, erythrocytes, occasionally leucocytes, and tissue debris.

— The nucleus is spherical in shape, 4-7 μm in size, and contains a central karyosome surrounded by a clear halo, anchored to the nuclear membrane by fine radiating fibrils known as the linin network, giving a wheel-like appearance.

— The nucleus is not clearly visible in living trophozoites but can be demonstrated in preparations stained with iron-hematoxylin.

— The nuclear membrane is lined by a rim of chromatin distributed evenly as small granules.

— Trophozoites from acute dysenteric stools often contain phagocytosed erythrocytes, a diagnostic feature not found in any other commensal intestinal amoebae.

溶组织内阿米巴滋养体内质着色较深，外质着色较浅，两者分界清晰，内质中除含细胞核外还有红细胞，核仁较小，常位于中央，核周染色质粒大小均匀、排列整齐。

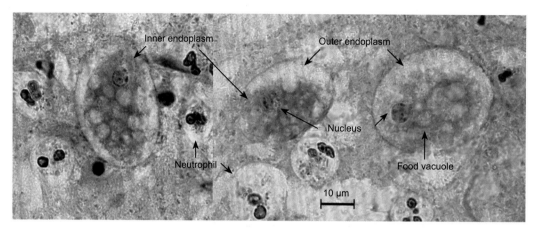

Figure 6-1　Trophozoites of *E. histolytica*

(2) Cysts of *E. histolytica* (Iron-hematoxylin stain) (Figure 6-2)

— Spherical in shape, approximately 10-16 μm in size.

— Early cysts contain a single nucleus, a mass of glycogen, and 1-4 chromatoid bodies or chromidial bars.

— The chromatoid bodies are cigar-shaped refractile rods with rounded ends, staining with hematoxylin (e.g. chromatin) .

— The nucleus in mature cyst undergoes 2 successive mitotic divisions, resulting in 2 and then 2 nuclei, making the mature cyst quadrinucleate.

— As the cyst matures, the glycogen mass and chromidial bars disappear.

— With iron-hematoxylin stain, the nuclear chromatin and chromatoid bodies appear deep blue or black, while the glycogen mass remains unstained.

— When stained with iodine, the glycogen mass appears golden brown, the nuclear chromatin and karyosome appear bright yellow, and the chromatoid bodies appear as clear space, remaining unstained.

　　溶组织内阿米巴包囊呈圆形，囊壁不着色。细胞质为灰蓝色致密颗粒状。细胞核结构与滋养体相同。染成深蓝色的拟染色体多呈棒状，两端钝圆。糖原块被溶解，仅留空泡状的痕迹，称为糖原泡。成熟包囊内含有4个细胞核。

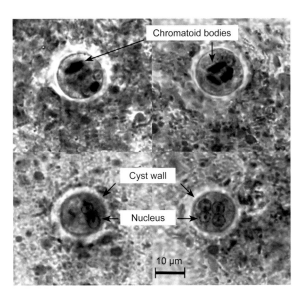

Figure 6-2　Cysts of *E. histolytica*

(3) Trophozoites and cysts of *E. coli* (Iron-hematoxylin stain)

— The morphology of *E. coli* is very similar to *E. histolytica*.

— The trophozoites are larger than *E. histolytica*, measuring approximately 15-50 μm. The nucleus is clearly visible and has a large eccentric karyosome and thick nuclear membrane (Figure 6-3) .

— The cysts are large, ranging from 10-35 μm in size. In the early stage, they exhibit a prominent glycogen mass. The chromatoid bodies are splinter-like and irregular. The mature cyst contains 8 nuclei (Figure 6-4) .

Key point

结肠内阿米巴包囊呈圆形或类圆形，比溶组织内阿米巴包囊大，细胞核结构与滋养体相同，有时可见束草状或碎片状、两端尖细不齐，染成深蓝色的拟染色体，囊壁不着色。成熟包囊含8个细胞核。

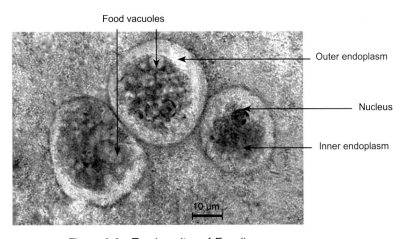

Figure 6-3　Trophozoites of *E. coli*

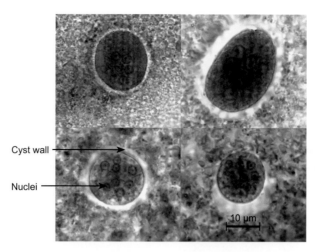

Figure 6-4　Cysts of *E. coli*

(4) Trophozoites of *G. lamblia* (Iron-hematoxylin stain) (Figure 6-5)

— The trophozoites have a rounded anterior and a pointed posterior, resembling the shape of a tennis racket or pyriform.

— Bilaterally symmetrical in shape.

— Measuring 15 μm long × 9 μm wide and 4 μm thick.

— They have convex dorsal surface and a concave sucking disc on the ventral side, aiding in their adhesion to the intestinal mucosa.

— Each cell contains 1 pair of nuclei, 4 pairs of flagella, 1 pair of median bodies, and 1 pair of axostyles running along the midline. Additionally, 2 sausage-shaped parabasal or median bodies locate transversely posterior to the sucking disc.

> **Key point**
>
> 　　蓝氏贾第鞭毛虫滋养体虫体呈梨形，前端宽圆，后端狭尖，前端腹面可见2个吸盘内各有一泡状核，前、腹、后、尾可见4对鞭毛。

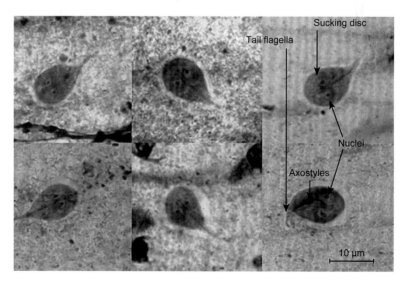

Figure 6-5　Trophozoites of *G. lamblia*

(5) Cysts of *G. lamblia* (Iron-hematoxylin stain) (Figure 6-6)

— Small and oval in shape.

— Measuring 8-14 μm in length and 7-10 μm in width.

— Surrounded by a hyaline cyst wall.

— The young cyst contains 1 pair of nuclei, while the mature cyst includes 2 pairs of nuclei grouped at one end.

— The axostyle lies diagonally, forming a dividing line on the cyst wall.

— Remnants of the flagella and the sucking disc may be observed in the young cyst.

Notes

> **Key point**
>
> 蓝氏贾第鞭毛虫包囊呈椭圆形，囊壁厚，不着色，泡状核位于包囊一端，成熟包囊含4个核。细胞质可见中体和鞭毛的早期结构。

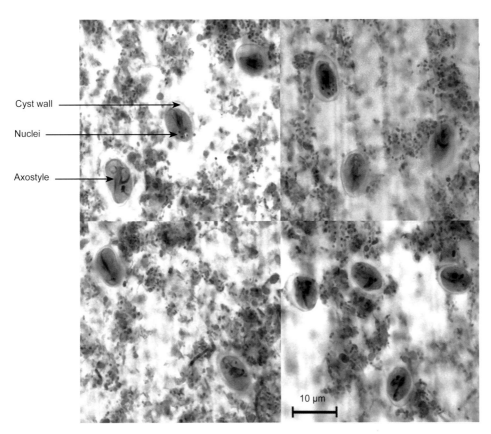

Figure 6-6　Cysts of *G. lamblia*

(6) Trophozoites of *T. vaginalis* (Giemsa or Wright's stain) (Figure 6-7)

— *Trichomonas* exists only in the trophozoite stage.

— Cystic stage is not observed.

— Pear or ovoid-shaped.

— Measuring 10-30 μm in length and 10-15 μm in breadth.

— They have a short undulating membrane that reaches up to the middle of the body.

— They have four anterior flagella and a fifth flagellum running along the outer margin of the undulating membrane (波动膜), which is supported by a flexible rod at its base called costa.

— A prominent axostyle runs throughout the length of the body and projects posteriorly like a tail.

— A large, ellipsoid nucleus is stained deep red and located adjacent to the anterior.

— The conspicuous siderophilic (嗜铁) granules known as hydrogenase body can be observed in the cytoplasm, which is most abundant alongside with the axostyle and costa.

> **Key point**
>
> 阴道毛滴虫滋养体虫体多为梨形，前端可见4根鞭毛，波动膜在虫体一侧，较短，一般不超过虫体一半，轴柱贯穿虫体并从末端伸出。细胞核在虫体前1/3处，呈椭圆形，核内具有分布均匀的染色质，细胞质内具有染色质粒，多分布在轴柱两侧。

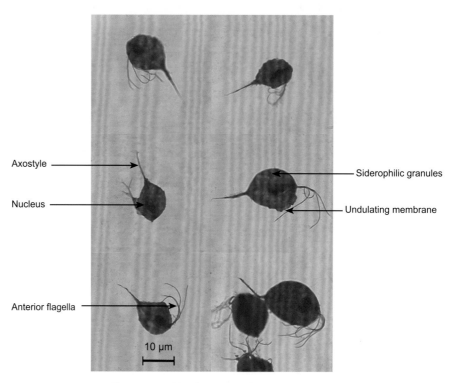

Figure 6-7　Trophozoites of *T. vaginalis*

Notes

2. *L. donovani* (under oil immersion lens)

(1) Amastigote (Giemsa, or Wright's stain, Figure 6-8)

— The amastigote form is also referred to as the LD body when observed under a microscope.

— It is very tiny, measuring 2.9-5.7 μm in size and 1.8-4.0 μm in width under the oil immersion lens.

— Ovoid or rounded in shape.

— They are found typically intracellularly inside macrophages, monocytes, neutrophils, or endothelial cells.

— The cytoplasm is pale blue and enclosed by a thin membrane.

— The large oval nucleus is stained red.

— The small kinetoplast near the nucleus is stained red or purple.

— In well-stained preparations, the kinetoplast can be observed consisting of a parabasal body and a dot-like blepharoplast with a fine thread connecting the two. The axoneme arising from the blepharoplast extends to the anterior tip of the cell. A clear unstained vacuole can be observed alongside the kinetoplast.

— It lacks a flagellum.

— Please note the differences between the LD body and blood platelets in the smear.

Key point

杜氏利什曼原虫无鞭毛体(利杜体)为圆形或椭圆形的小体，常在吞噬细胞内或游离于细胞之外。大小仅为红细胞的1/3，细胞质染为蓝色，较大的胞核染成紫红色，在细胞核旁可见一杆状红色小点，即动基体。

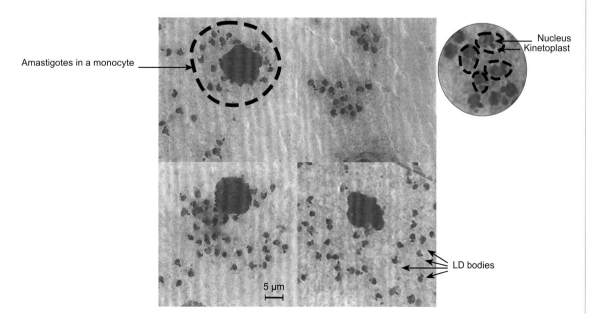

Figure 6-8　Amastigotes of *L. donovani*

(2) Promastigote (Giemsa stain, Figure 6-9)

— It is a flagellar stage and can be seen in insect vector, sandfly and in culture.

— The promastigotes begin as short, oval or pear-shaped forms, and later develop into long spindle shaped cells that are 15-20 μm long and 1.5-3.5 μm wide.

— A prominent nucleus is situated at the center. The kinetoplast lies transversely near the anterior end.

— The flagellum is single, delicate, and measures 15-28 μm, the same as the cell length.

— Giemsa or Wright-stained films show pale blue cytoplasm with a pink nucleus and bright red kinetoplast.

— A vacuole may be present near the root of the flagellum.

— There is no undulating membrane.

Key point

　　杜氏利什曼原虫前鞭毛体呈狭长纺锤状，前端钝圆尾端尖细。细胞核位于中央，染为红色，细胞质呈蓝色，红色的鞭毛自虫体前端发出，长度等于或超过体长。

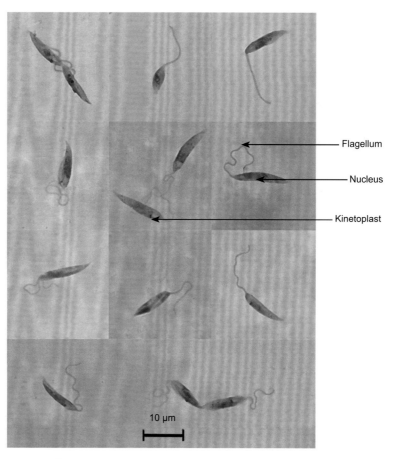

Figure 6-9　Promastigotes of *L. donovani*

3. Histopathological sections of intestinal amoebiasis (H & E stain, Figure 6-10)

— A cross-section through a colon ulcer reveals the formation of superficial ulceration.

— The invasive trophozoites cause lysis of the mucosal epithelium in areas where the mucus layer is depleted.

— These lesions are most commonly found in the cecum, appendix, or ascending portion of colon, deeply involving in the lamina propria and submucosa.

— The distinctive flask-shaped ulcers are formed as trophozoites expand laterally in these layers.

— In the typical lesion, erosion of the mucosal epithelium extends to the muscularis. Numerous trophozoites and inflammatory cells are observed in the section through a colon ulcer.

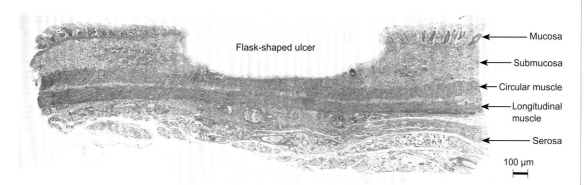

Figure 6-10   Section of mucosa suffered from intestinal amoebiasis

Notes

Demonstrations on the display bench

1. Colon mucosa involved with intestinal amoebiasis

Amoebic ulcer is the typical lesion seen in the colon. The ulcers are multiple and confined to the colon, with the highest number in the cecum and the second highest in the sigmoid-rectal region. The intervening mucosa membrane between the ulcers remains healthy. The ulcers appear initially on the mucosa as raised nodules with pouting edges, which later break down and discharge brownish necrotic material containing large numbers of trophozoites. The typical amoebic ulcer is flask-shaped in cross section, with a narrow mouth and neck, and a large and rounded base (Figure 6-11) .

> **Key point**
>
> 肠阿米巴病理标本可见肠壁溃疡呈散在性分布，大小不一，病变中央组织缺损，周围组织水肿而隆起，形成"火山口"样。多个溃疡融合后，使肠黏膜组织坏死、脱落，形成浅表溃疡。溃疡口小底大，溃疡之间仍可见到正常组织。

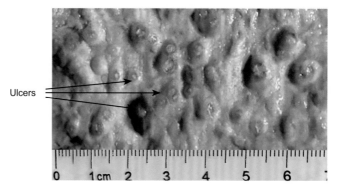

Figure 6-11   Gross view of amoebic ulcers

2. Histopathological sections of intestinal amoebiasis (H & E stain, under high power lens)

Numerous trophozoites of *E. histolytica* enter the lamina propria of mucosa, with countless inflammatory cells infiltrating the lesion. The nuclei of the oval trophozoites can be observed as small, darker-staining circles within the cytoplasm of the amebae. The empty region around the trophozoites reflects amebae shrinking during the fixation process (Figure 6-12) .

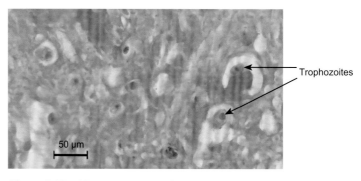

Figure 6-12   Mucosal section of intestinal amoebiasis

Notes

Practices

1. Draw trophozoites of *E. histolytica*, *G. lamblia*, *T. vaginalis*, and a promastigote of *L. donovani*.
2. Draw mature cysts of *E. histolytica* and *G. lamblia*.
3. Outline the life cycle of *L. donovani* with short text and arrows.

Quiz

1. Which one is the trophozoites of *E. histolytica*?

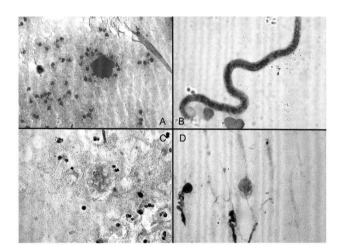

2. Which one is the promastigotes of *L. donovani*?

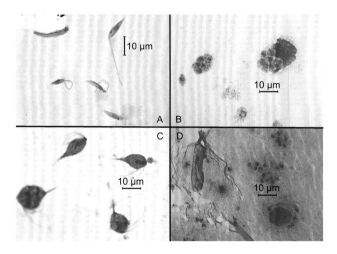

Notes

3. Which one is mature cysts of *G. lamblia*?

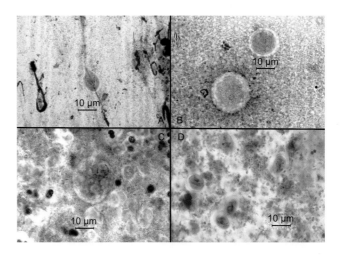

4. How to diagnose the intestinal lesion and the exo-intestinal lesion of *E. histolytica*?

5. Why people infected with *G. lamblia* suffer diarrhea?

Case analysis

Case 1

A 22-year-old female presented to the local hospital with symptoms of abdominal pain, cramps and diarrhea. She reported recently returning from a trip to Vietnam. Stool samples were collected and preserved in 10% formalin and polyvinyl alcohol (PVA) for O & P testing. Figure 6-13 depicts the findings observed at 1000× magnification on iron-hematoxylin-stained slide prepared from the PVA-preserved feces. The observed structures had an average diameter of 15-17 micrometers. Based on these findings, what is your medical diagnosis?

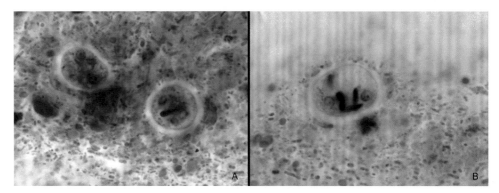

Figure 6-13   Typical objects observed under microscope

Notes

Case 2

A 35-year-old female presented to the hospital with ulcerative sores on her left ear and neck. Four months prior, she had traveled along the Amazon River in Brazil, where she also experienced multiple insect bites. The patient was referred to an infectious disease specialist, who obtained a biopsy sample from the largest lesion. The sample was sent to the Pathological laboratory for sectioning and staining with Giemsa. Figure 6-14 illustrates the findings at a magnification of 1000×. What is your medical diagnosis? Would you recommend any further examinations for an accurate diagnosis?

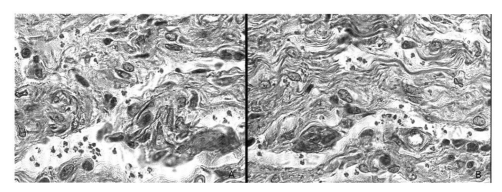

Figure 6-14   Typical views of the sample under microscope

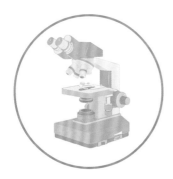

Practice 7　Protozoa II

Classification

Plasmodium (疟原虫)
　　Plasmodium vivax (间日疟原虫, 间日疟)
　　Plasmodium falciparum (恶性疟原虫, 恶性疟)
　　Plasmodium malariae (三日疟原虫, 三日疟)
　　Plasmodium ovale (卵形疟原虫, 卵形疟)
Toxoplasma gondii (弓形虫)
Babesia (巴贝虫)

◎ Objectives

1. Identify all blood stages of *P. vivax*, the ring stage and gametocyte stages of *P. falciparum*, and the tachyzoites of *T. gondii*.
2. Practice at least one time for preparing both thin and thick blood smears for malaria testing and making a blood smear of *P. berghei*.
3. Describe the morphology of *Babesia* species.

Observations

1. All blood stages of *P. vivax* (Giemsa stain, under oil immersion lens)

(1) Early trophozoite (ring form, Figure 7-1)

— The ring form refers to the ring-like appearance of the malaria parasite following invading into a previously healthy red blood cell.

— The typical ring is well-defined, with a blue cytoplasmic circle, a prominent central vacuole, and a red chromatin dot (nucleus).

— One side of the ring is thicker, while the other side is thinner.

— The nucleus is situated on the thin side.

— The ring is approximately 2.5-3.0 μm in diameter, about a third of the size of an erythrocyte.

Key point

　　疟原虫的小滋养体（环状体）呈指环状，细胞质为蓝色、环形，包围糖原空泡。细胞核呈红色点状，位于环的一侧。原虫约占红细胞直径的1/3，形似红宝石戒指。被疟原虫感染的红细胞不胀大。薛氏小点与疟色素还不可见。

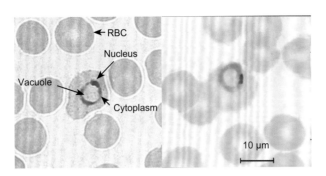

Figure 7-1   Ring forms of *P. vivax*

(2) Trophozoite (Figure 7-2)

— The ring develops rapidly to an amoeboid form parasite after approximately 10 hours of growth in erythrocyte.

— The cytoplasm of the parasite stains light blue, while the nucleus stains red or rose red.

— The vacuole remains visible and basically intact until the late stage of development.

— Hemozoin pigment granules, primary dark brown in color, become apparent in the cytoplasm and increase in amount and visibility as the parasites mature.

— Infected erythrocytes enlarge and display red granules known as Schüffner's dots on their surface. They become irregular in shape, lose their red color, and appear washed-out.

Key point

　　大滋养体期疟原虫形态变化较大，呈不规则的阿米巴形，疟色素在细胞质内呈黄褐色烟末状。细胞核稍粗大，但没有分裂。被寄生的红细胞开始胀大，红细胞膜表面可见红色颗粒状的薛氏小点(Schüffner's dots)。

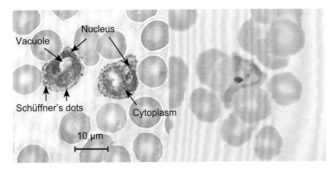

Figure 7-2   Trophozoites of *P. vivax*

(3) Immature schizont (Figure 7-3)

— The cytoplasmic material is more abundant but still unseparated.

— The nucleus starts to divide into multiple chromatin bodies, which stain as red dots.

— Hemozoin is widely distributed in the cytoplasm of the parasite.

Key point

　　未成熟裂殖体的细胞质内疟色素呈烟丝状，细胞核开始分裂，但细胞质无分裂。细胞核数目在2个以上，其他均与大滋养体相同。

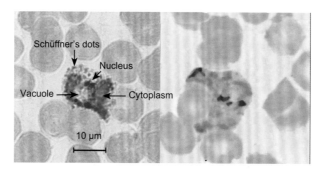

Figure 7-3　Immature schizonts of *P. vivax*

(4) Mature schizont (Figure 7-4)

— The schizont appears approximately 36-40 hours after invasion.

— Continued division of chromatin results in 14 to 24 (usually 16) individual merozoites.

— These merozoites, surrounded by cytoplasmic material, occupy almost the entire enlarged red blood cell.

— Malaria pigment aggregates as small brownish dots.

Key point

　　成熟裂殖体核分裂为12～24个，细胞质也分裂并包裹在核的周围，形成12～24个裂殖子，裂殖子排列不规则。疟色素与残存的细胞质形成残余体，常位于原虫的一侧，被寄生的红细胞明显胀大。

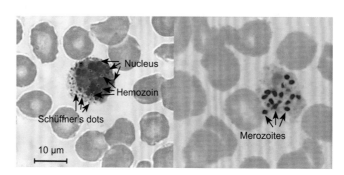

Figure 7-4　Mature schizonts of *P. vivax*

(5) Gametocyte (Figure 7-5, Figure 7-6)

— Gametocytes appear early, usually within 4 days after the trophozoites first appear.

— Both male (microgametocyte) and female (macrogametocyte) are large, nearly fill the enlarged red blood cell.

— The female gametocyte has dense cytoplasm that stains deep blue and a small, compact, eccentric nucleus, often located against the edge of the parasite. Delicate, diffuse, light brown pigment may be visible throughout the parasite.

— The male gametocyte has pale-staining (even colorless) cytoplasm and a large, diffuse, pink/purple nucleus residing the center. The pigment granules are prominent and dispersive.

> **Key point**
>
> 雌、雄配子体虫体近球形，有一个细胞核，细胞质染成蓝色，边缘整齐，内无空泡，其中散布有棕色疟色素颗粒。细胞核与细胞质之间常有不染色的空白带。雌配子体较大，常大于正常的红细胞，故又称大配子体，细胞质颜色较深，核较小，其核内颗粒排列致密，故色深，位于细胞一侧。雄配子体常较正常的红细胞小，故又称小配子体，细胞质颜色较浅，核内颗粒排列疏松，故色浅，多位于细胞中心。

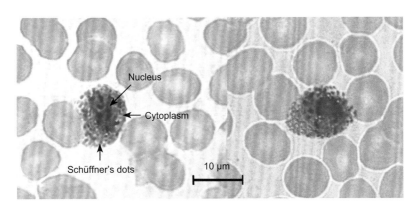

Figure 7-5 Microgametocytes of *P. vivax*

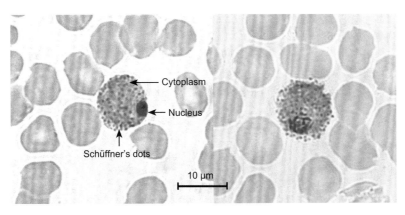

Figure 7-6 Macrogametocytes of *P. vivax*

Notes

2. Major blood stages of *P. falciparum* (Giemsa stain, under oil immersion lens)

(1) Ring form (Figure 7-7)

— Measuring 1.5 μm in diameter, and approximately one-fifth (1/5) the size of a red blood cell.

— It consists of minimal cytoplasm connected to one or two small nuclei.

— Binucleate rings (double chromatin) commonly resembles stereo headphones in appearance.

— Rings are often seen attached along the edge of the red blood cell.

— A small vacuole is usually visible within the parasite.

— Multiple rings within a single red blood cell are frequently observed.

Key point

恶性疟原虫的小滋养体较纤细，直径约为红细胞直径的1/5，偶有2个细胞核。一个红细胞内可有2个或2个以上的疟原虫寄生。

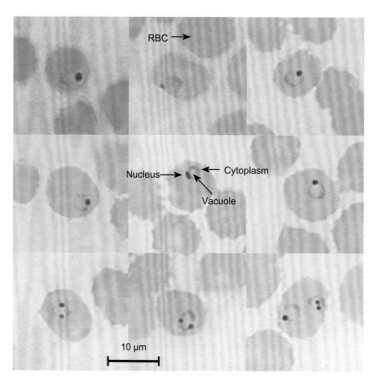

Figure 7-7   Ring forms of *P. falciparum*

(2) Gametocyte (Figure 7-8, Figure 7-9)

— Gametocytes appear in circulation about 10 days after the initial appearance of the ring stage.

— Mature gametocytes observed in peripheral smears are curved oblong structures, described as crescentic, sickle, sausage, or banana-shaped. They are usually referred to as crescents.

— Male gametocytes are broad and sausage-shaped or kidney-shaped, with blunt rounded ends as compared to the females.

— Female gametocytes are thinner and more typically crescentic, with sharply rounded or pointed ends.

— The cytoplasm of female gametocyte stains deep blue, while in males it appears pale blue or pink.

— The nucleus of female gametocytes is compact and stains deep red, with the pigment granules closely aggregated around it. In males, it is pink, large and diffuse, with scattered pigment granules in the cytoplasm.

— Mature gametocytes are longer than the diameter of a red blood cell, causing gross distortion and sometimes apparent disappearance of the infected red blood cell.

— The membrane red blood cell is often seen as a rim on the concave side of the gametocyte.

Notes

Key point

　　雌配子体呈新月形，虫体两端较尖，细胞质为蓝色，红色的细胞核位于虫体中部，棕色的颗粒状或短棒状的疟色素散布于虫体或核的周围。雄配子体为香蕉形，虫体两端钝圆，细胞质为淡蓝色，红色的细胞核位于虫体中部，色较雌配子体浅，棕色的颗粒状或短棒状的疟色素散布于虫体或细胞核的周围。

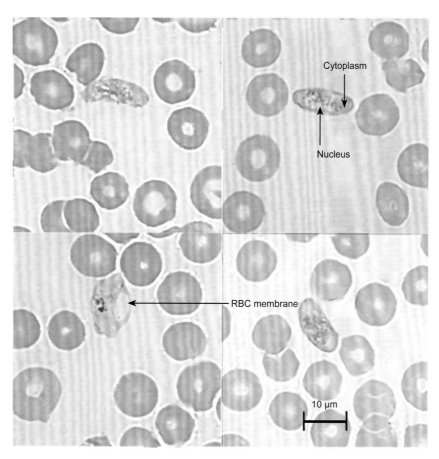

Figure 7-8　Microgametocytes of *P. falciparum*

(3) Trophozoite, immature schizont, mature schizont (Figure 7-10)

— These forms are not commonly observed in the peripheral blood unless the patient is severely infected.

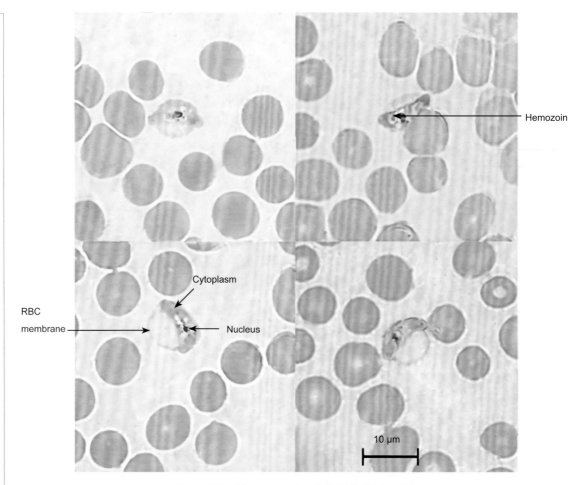

Figure 7-9   Macrogametocytes of *P. falciparum*

— The presence of *P. falciparum* schizonts in peripheral smears indicates a grave prognosis.

— These forms resemble the same stage of *P. vivax*. The infected red blood cells are not significantly larger than those infected with *P. vivax*. The pigments in the parasite cytoplasm often aggregate together. Coarse blue or dark blue Maurer's dots (茂氏点) are apparent on the surface of erythrocytes at the trophozoite stage.

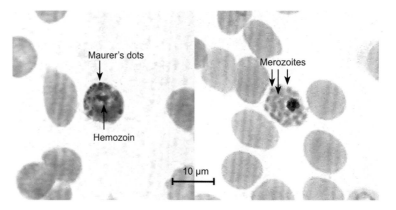

Figure 7-10   Trophozoite (left) and schizont (right) of *P. falciparum*

3. Tachyzoites of *T. gondii* (Giemsa stain, Figure 7-11)

— The trophozoites are crescent-shaped, with one end pointed and the other end rounded.

— They measure 4-7 μm in length and 2-4 μm in width.

— The cytoplasm stains light blue

— The red nucleus is ovoid and situated at the blunt end of the parasites.

Notes

Key point

　　弓形虫速殖子呈弓形或新月形，一端较钝圆，一端较尖细。细胞质呈蓝色，细胞核呈红色。

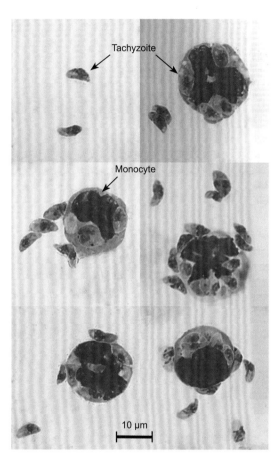

Figure 7-11　Tachyzoites of *T. gondii*

4. *B. microti* (Giemsa stain)

— Trophozoites are polymorphic, measuring 2-5 μm in diameter, and are found inside the red blood cells.

— They may have a pyriform, amoeboid, or spindle-like shape, often appearing in pairs and sometimes mistaken for the ring form of *Plasmodium*.

— Merozoites may be spherical, oval, or pyriform bodies, found in pairs, forming a "Maltese cross". Babesia does not generate hemozoin in the infected red blood cells (Figure 7-12) .

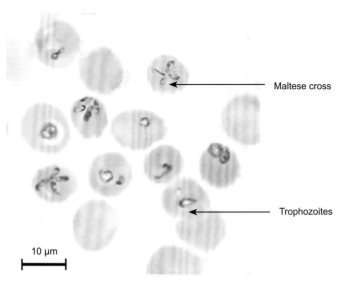

Figure 7-12   Different stages of *B. microti*

Demonstrations on the display bench

1. Oocysts of *T. gondii*

They are round to slightly oval, measuring 10 to 15 μm in length and 8 to 12 μm in width. The transparent oocyst contains two sporocysts, each with four sporozoites. The organism is surrounded by a clear, colorless, two-layered cell wall (Figure 7-13) .

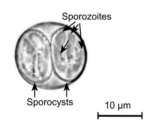

Figure 7-13   Oocyst of *T. gondii*

2. Oocysts of *P. Vivax*

Oocysts of *Plasmodium* species reside on the stomach wall of mosquito: Numerous oval or elliptic oocysts stain dark blue. The sporozoites within the oocyst cannot be identified (Figure 7-14) .

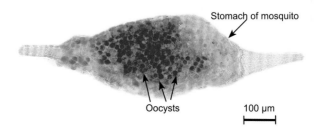

Figure 7-14   Oocysts of *P. vivax* on the stomach wall of a mosquito (Wright's stain)

3. Sporozoites of *Plasmodium* species (Smear)

The sporozoites measure 10-15 μm in length. They are single nucleated, spindle shaped with equally pointed ends. The sporozoites are the infective form found in infected mosquitoes and are infectious to human (Figure 7-15) .

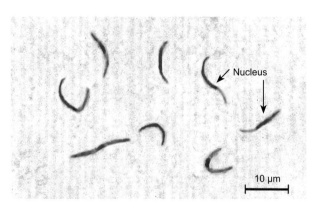

Figure 7-15   Sporozoites of *P. falciparum*

Practices

1. Preparation of a thin blood smear of *P. berghei*

1) Making the thin blood smear

— Collect one drop of blood from the scissor-cut tail of infected mice and place it on one end of a clean slide.

— Contact the drop with the long edge of another slide and hold it at an angle of 30°-45° against the bottom-slide.

— Move the top-slide directing towards the other end of the bottom-slide to make a thin and uniform smear.

— Air dry the smear. The thickness will depend on the size of the drop, the angle between the slides, and the speed of movement.

2) Fixing: Fix the dried thin film by covering it with several drops of methyl alcohol and allow it to air dry.

3) Giemsa stain

— Cover the smear with 2% Giemsa's solution (working solution) and keep it for 15 min.

— Wash the smear by pouring neutral distilled water over the slide until the dyeing solution completely washed away.

— Drain the slide and stand on one end to dry.

4) Observation: Examine the slide under oil immersion lens (Figure 7-16) .

2. Dissection of mouse model infected with *T. gondii*

1) Sacrifice the mice with one week-post infection and explore the peritoneal cavity (Figure 7-17 A). Observe the pathological enlargement of liver, spleen (Figure 7-17 B) .

2) Prepare a Giemsa-stained thin blood smear to observe the tachyzoites of *T. gondii* under oil immersion lens (Figure 7-17 C) .

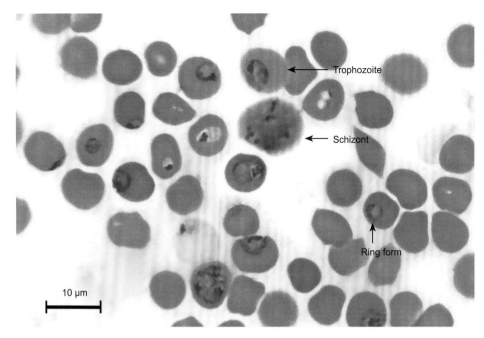

Figure 7-16   Blood smear of *P. berghei* infected mouse under microscope

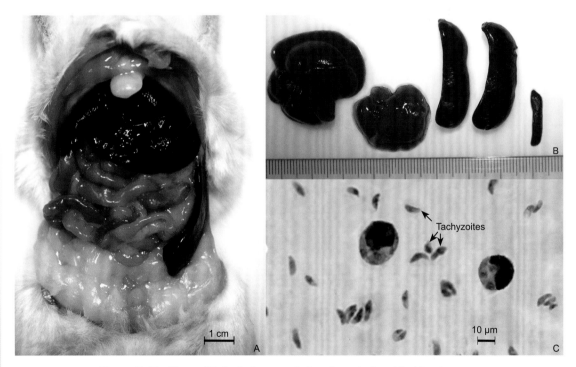

Figure 7-17   *T. gondii* infected mouse being dissected and its blood smear

3. Draw all blood stages of *P. vivax*, the ring stage and both genders of gametocytes of *P. falciparum*, and the tachyzoite of *T. gondii*.

4. Outline the life cycle of *T. gondii* using words, short sentences, and arrows.

Quiz

1. Which one is the trophozoite of *P. vivax*?

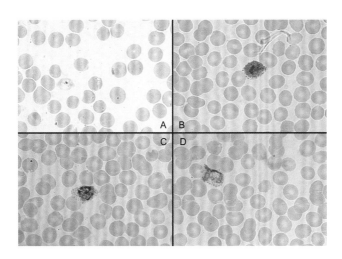

2. Which one is the male gametocyte of *P. plasmodium*?

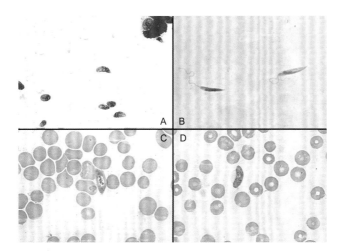

3. Compare the life cycles of *P. vivax* and *P. falciparum*, find out their differences and discuss the relevance of these differences to pathogenesis, diagnosis, and prevalence.

4. Explain the phenomenon of paroxysm, recrudescence and relapse based on the life cycles of *Plasmodium* species.

Case analysis

Case 1

A 45-year-old male patient who frequently travels worldwide for business and has recently commuted among Myanmar, China and South Korea. He presented with a two-week history of low-grade fever and no other symptoms. A blood smear was taken and examined at the hospital laboratory. Figure 7-18 shows the findings on one of the thin smears. What is your diagnosis? Where do you think he contracted the disease?

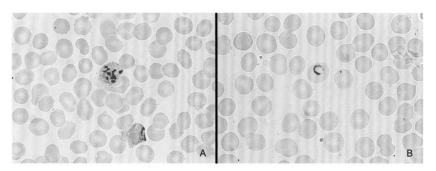

Figure 7-18 Typical objects observed under microscope

Case 2

A 25-year-old Chinese woman recently completed a two-month trip to several countries in West Africa. She chose chloroquine for malaria prevention, although she was not fully adherent to this regimen. She stopped taking the medicine halfway through her vacation due to stomach discomfort. After returning to China three days later, she developed a high-grade fever (39.1°C) and chills but no respiratory symptoms such as cough or runny nose. She had a normal appetite and no vomiting, diarrhea, or jaundice. Considering her recent travel history in West African, thin blood smears were taken and stained for malaria diagnosis. Figure 7-19 shows the specimen stained with Wright stain. What is your diagnosis? Based on what criteria?

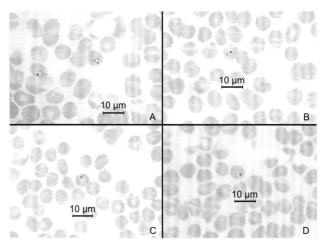

Figure 7-19 Typical objects observed under microscope

Notes

Case 3

An elderly man with a fever, nausea, abdominal pain, and general weakness visited the doctor. He had not traveled outside of the United States in the past 5 years. However, he mentioned being bitten by a black-bug on his farm recently. Based on his clinical presentation, the symptoms were presumed to be related to bug bites. A blood smear stained with Giemsa was requested and examined. Figure 7-20 displays the findings on the stained smears. What has been observed? Please share your opinion.

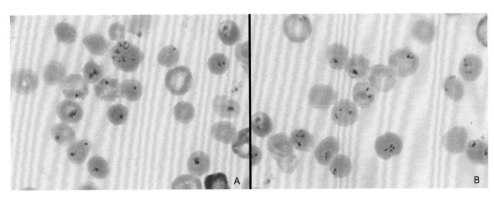

Figure 7-20   Typical objects observed under microscope

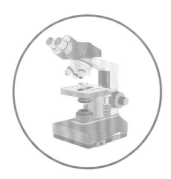

Practice 8　Medical arthropods

Classification

Mosquito (蚊)

Fly (蝇)

Sandfly (白蛉)

Flea (蚤)

Louse (虱)

Bedbug (臭虫)

Tick (蜱)

Chigger mite (恙螨)

Scab mite (疥螨)

Demodicid mite (蠕形螨)

◎ Objectives

1. Describe the characteristics of mosquitoes, flies, sand fly, fleas, lice, ticks and mites.
2. Distinguish between hard ticks and soft ticks based on their morphology.

Observations

1. Adult mosquitoes (Figure 8-1)

— The body consists of 3 segments: head, thorax, and abdomen.

— The head is roundish and connected to the elongate thorax by a slender neck.

— The abdomen is also elongated and comprises 10 segments.

— Only 8 of the abdominal segments are usually visible.

— A single pair of antennae is long and has 15 segments.

— Three pairs of legs extend from the thorax region.

— Mosquitoes have 2 pairs of wings, with 1 pair smaller than the other.

— The size of mosquitoes varies depending on the species.

— The Anopheles mosquito, for example, generally measures 6 to 8 mm long.

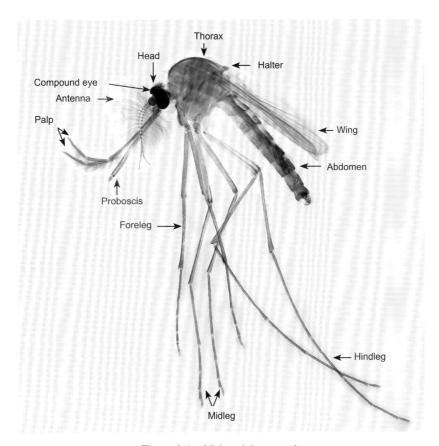

Figure 8-1   Male adult mosquito

2. Adult Flies (Figure 8-2).

— All species possess 2 pairs of wings.

— One pair is smaller than the other.

— The head, thorax, and segmented abdomen appear as 3 separate sections.

— Flies have 1 pair of antennae, 1 pair of eyes, and 3 pairs of legs.

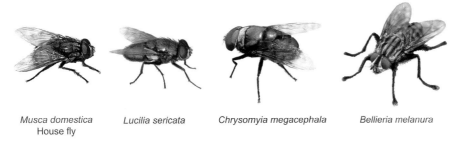

Musca domestica   *Lucilia sericata*   *Chrysomyia megacephala*   *Bellieria melanura*
House fly

Figure 8-2   Adult flies

3. Adult sandfly (Figure 8-3)
— Brown-yellow in body color and fully hairy.
— They have 1 pair of relatively large black eyes.
— Three pairs of long legs.
— The wings are held erect over the body, giving the fly an angel-like appearance.

Key point

　　白蛉成虫较蚊体小，棕黄色，全身披毛，头部有一对较大的眼，胸部向背面隆起，似驼背，翅窄长而尖，静止时双翅向背侧展开。

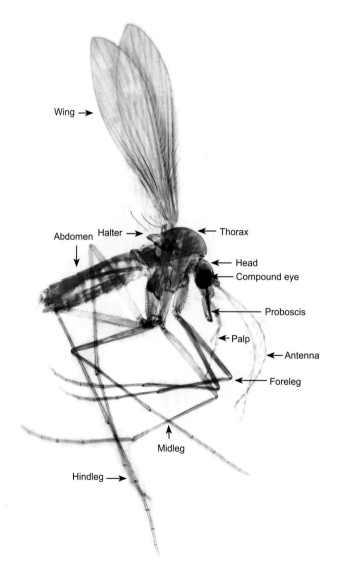

Figure 8-3　Female adult sandfly

4. Adult Flea (Figure 8-4)

— Small wingless insects of the order *Siphonaptera*, ranging from 1.3 to 4 mm in size.

— They have 3 pairs of powerful hairy legs with claw-like feet, and the rear pair of legs is extralong, enable them to move quickly by jumping.

— Their small and segmented bodies are flattened from side to side, allowing them to move through their hosts' feathers or hair.

— Their mouthparts are specialized for piercing and blood-sucking.

— The presence or absence of eyes, the mouthparts (called genal ctenidia，颊栉）, and pronotal ctenidia (前胸栉, comb-like structures located closely behind the head and extending posteriorly on the flea's dorsal side) aid in the differentiation of flea species.

Notes

> **Key point**
>
> 蚤成虫体呈黄褐色，分节，短小，两侧稍扁平，全身有许多向后生长的鬃和刺，有些蚤的颊部和前胸后缘有黑色坚硬粗壮的刺，称为颊栉或前胸栉。

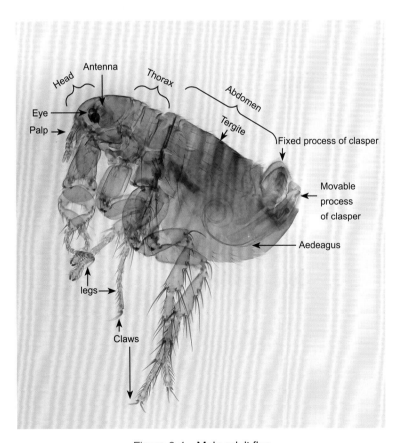

Figure 8-4   Male adult flea

Notes

5. Adult louse (Figure 8-5)

— Wingless, with flattened bodies.

— Three pairs of legs, with large claws at the end for clinging onto hair.

— Three different kinds of lice have been found on the human body: head lice (*Pediculus humanus capitis*) , body lice (*Pediculus humanus corporis*) , and pubic lice (*Phthirus pubis,* 耻阴虱) .

— Head lice have a head, thorax and abdomen with 6 legs. They are commonly grey-white in color.

— Pubic lice are commonly called "crabs" due to their resemblance to a crab.

> **Key point**
>
> 虱成虫呈灰白色或灰色，体、背、腹扁平，分头、胸、腹三部。头略呈锥形，黑眼一对，具有刺吸式口器，足三对，短，跗节末端有一爪与胫节末端的胫突相对形成攫握器，可紧握宿主的头发或衣服纤维。

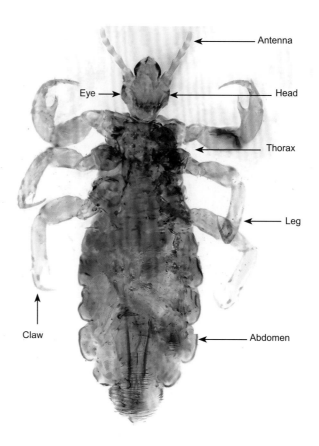

Figure 8-5   Adult body louse

6. Adult bedbug (Figure 8-6)

— The adult bedbugs are 5-7 mm long and 4-5 mm wide, similar in size to an apple seed.

— They have a flat, oval-shaped body, brown or reddish-brown in color.

— A beak with three segments.

— Antennae consist of four parts.

— Wings are not used for flying.

— The entire body is covered by short, golden-colored hairs.

— They emit a distinct "musty-sweetish" odor produced by glands on the lower side of their body.

Notes

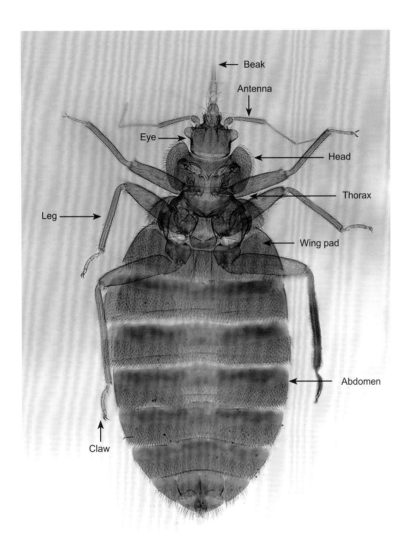

Figure 8-6   Adult bedbug

Notes

7. Adult hard and soft ticks (Figure 8-7, Figure 8-8, Table 8-1)

— Typical ticks range from 6 to 8 mm long in size.

— Adult ticks have 4 pairs of legs, 2 pairs of mouthparts, and no antennae.

— Both male and female ticks have an oval shape.

— The head and thorax are fused into cephalothorax (头 胸 部), which is connected to the abdominal region together as a single structure.

— Hard ticks have a visible capitulum (假头, a term referring to the mouthparts of ticks and mites) on their dorsal side, while soft ticks have an invisible capitulum due to their ventral positioning.

— Hard ticks have a dorsal hard shield called chitinous scutum (盾板) located posterior to the capitulum, covering the entire dorsal surface in males and the anterior part in females.

— Soft ticks lack chitinous scutum and have a leathery outer surface.

Key point

硬蜱假头位于躯体前方，从背面可以看到雄虫盾板大，遮盖整个背面，雌虫盾板小，仅覆盖背部前侧，故雄虫、雌虫易区别。软蜱假头位于躯体腹面前方，从背面无法看到。软蜱无盾板，故雄虫、雌虫不易区别。

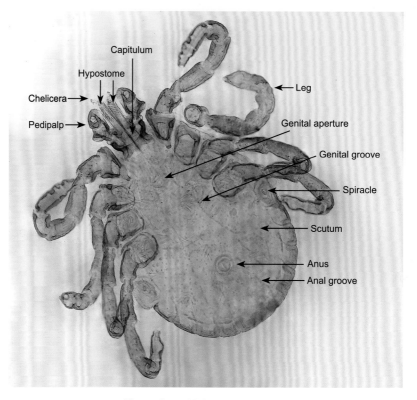

Figure 8-7　Male adult hard tick

Notes

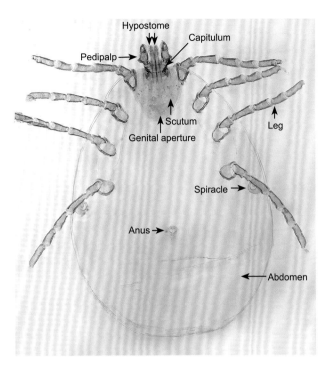

Figure 8-8   Female adult hard tick

Table 8-1   Hard and soft adult ticks: typical features at a glance

Characteristic	Hard ticks	Soft ticks
Fused spherical body (head, thorax, abdomen together)	√	√
4 pairs of legs	√	√
Visible capitulum on dorsal side	√	×
Capitulum on ventral side	√	√
Scutum	√	×

8. Adult scab mites (*Sarcoptes scabiei*, 疥螨) (Figure 8-9)

— Small, measuring 0.3-0.5 mm, but still visible to the naked eye.

— Oval in shape.

— The dorsal surface of the body is scattered with transverse ridges (横纹), spines (刺), and bristles(刚毛).

— The mouthparts consist of toothed chelicerae (螯肢).

— They have four pairs of short but stout legs.

— In males, the first two and the fourth pairs of legs terminate with claws and a bell-shaped sucker (ambulacra, 吸垫). The third pairs of legs end with long bristles (鬃).

— In females, claws and ambulacra are only seen in the first two pairs of legs, while the last two pairs of legs end with long bristles.

Key point

　　疥螨成虫虫体小，呈短椭圆形，背面有波状皱纹及长短不一的刚毛和刺，足4对，较短。雌雄成螨前两对足末端均有长柄吸垫，雌螨后两对足末端均长有长鬃，而雄螨只有第三对足末端长有长鬃，第四对足末端仍是具长柄的吸垫。

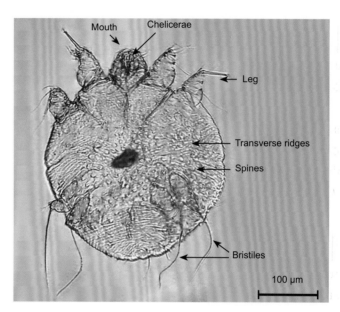

Figure 8-9　Adult female scab mite

9. Adult *Demodicid* mites (Figure 8-10)

— *Demodex folliculorum* (毛囊蠕形螨) and *Demodex brevis* (皮脂蠕形螨) are the only Demodicid mites found on humans.

— Both species primarily inhabit the area of the nose, forehead, and the eyebrows, but can also occur elsewhere on the body.

— Adult mites measure only 0.3-0.4 mm in length, with *D. folliculorum* slightly longer than *D. brevis*.

— They are semi-transparent, elongated, and cigar-shaped.

— Eight short segmented legs are attached to the anterior half of the body.

— The opisthosoma (末体) , the posterior of the body, is transversely striated.

Key point

　　蠕形螨成虫体长，呈蠕虫状，乳白色，躯体分足体和末体两部分，末体表有环状横纹。毛囊蠕形螨较长，足体约占体长的1/3，足4对，末体占体长的2/3。皮脂蠕形螨略短，足体约占体长的1/2。

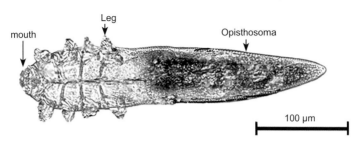

Figure 8-10　Adult *D. folliculorum*

Practices

Self-survey for the infection of *Demodicid* mites
— Clean the face before preparing the collection of mites and do not apply any creams during the examination.
— Paste the transparent adhesive tape around the nose or forehead where the mites commonly inhabit for about 8 hours or overnight.
— Take the tape off in the morning and stick it on the slide for observation.
— Observe *Demodicid* mites in the film and record the result of the examination.

Quiz

1. Which arbo-disease can be prevented by eliminating mosquitoes in the city?
2. What kind of diseases can fly cause or transmit?

Case analysis

Case 1

A lab in India received an arthropod specimen from a parent whose child had been suffering for about a week with rashes over his extremities and back. The patient was initially treated for the rashes, but they returned. An organism was captured and sent to the parasitology department for diagnostic assistance. Figure 8-11 shows the images after the organism was prepared on the slide. What is your identification? Based on what criteria? What is the public health importance, if any, of this organism?

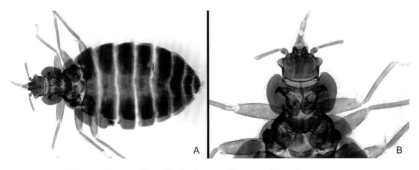

Figure 8-11　Detailed observations under microscope

Case 2

An old woman had been experiencing rashes on her arms and legs for about 3 months. The rashes were initially treated by the patient, but they kept coming back. She sent an arthropod specimen to the local clinic. The doctor received and made a slide for the specimen and observed some images of the organism under microscope. Figure 8-12 display two photos. What do you identify based on the morphology?

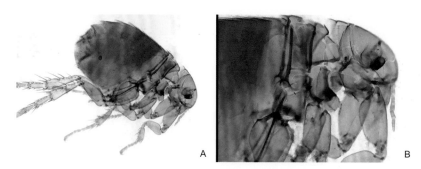

Figure 8-12　Detailed observation under microscope

Case 3

A Russian hunter came home from a weekend camping trip to find a tick adhered to his lower thigh. The parasitologist in local medical college was contacted for identification after the tick was extracted and taken to his medical laboratory. Figure 8-13 A depicts the tick's dorsal view. A close-up of the mouthparts is shown in Figure 8-13 B. Can you confirm the species of this tick? Based on what standards? What do you suggest to the hunter preventing from the ticks bite?

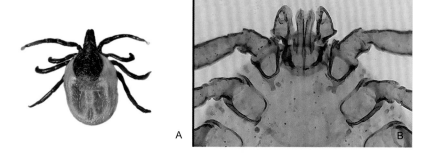

Figure 8-13　Detailed observations under microscope

Case 4

A 50 years old man from Yunnan province reported with rashes and pruritus on his chest. He mentioned that the symptoms remained for weeks despite regular washing. His breast hair was found to have possible arthropod ectoparasites (Figure 8-14 A) , therefore a specimen was obtained and submitted to the microbiological laboratory for analysis. A close-up image of the organisms under microscope was shown in Figure 8-14 B. The length of the thing was 1.5 mm. What is your diagnosis?

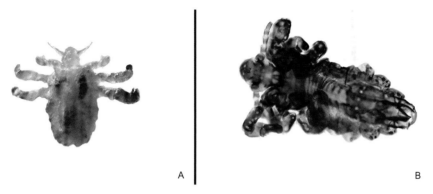

A   B

Figure 8-14   Detailed observations under microscope